# THINKING WOMEN
## AND HEALTH CARE REFORM
## IN CANADA

# THINKING WOMEN
## AND HEALTH CARE REFORM
## IN CANADA

edited by
**Pat Armstrong, Barbara Clow,
Karen Grant, Margaret Haworth-Brockman,
Beth Jackson, Ann Pederson,
and Morgan Seeley**

Women's Press
Toronto

*Thinking Women and Health Care Reform in Canada*
Pat Armstrong, Barbara Clow, Karen Grant, Margaret Haworth-Brockman, Beth Jackson, Ann Pederson and Morgan Seeley

First published in 2012 by
Women's Press, an imprint of Canadian Scholars' Press Inc.
180 Bloor Street West, Suite 801
Toronto, Ontario
M5S 2V6

www.womenspress.ca

Canadian Scholars' Press Inc./Women's Press gratefully acknowledges financial support for our publishing activities from the Government of Canada through the Canada Book Fund (CBF).

Library and Archives Canada Cataloguing in Publication

Thinking women and health care reform in Canada : international perspectives / Pat Armstrong ... [et al.].

Includes bibliographical references and index.
ISBN 978-0-88961-485-7

1. Women's health services—Canada. 2. Women caregivers—Canada. 3. Health care reform—Canada.
I. Armstrong, Pat, 1945–

RA564.85.T55 2012          362.1082          C2011-907293-9

Text design by Colleen Wormald
Cover design by Aldo Fierro

Printed and bound in Canada by Webcom

Canada

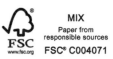

MIX
Paper from
responsible sources
FSC
www.fsc.org
FSC® C004071

# Table of Contents

# Introduction

PAT ARMSTRONG

There is no need to show Canadians that health care is a critical service and fundamental to our identity. Poll after poll indicates that health care is both our most valued social program and the issue of greatest concern for a majority. There is a need, however, to show Canadians that health care is an issue for women as a group and for particular groups of women, and to demonstrate that taking gender into account is essential for an effective health care system. This book is compiled by a unique group that, for more than a dozen years, has been seeking to address this need for a gender-based analysis of health care.

The group is unique because it is composed of members who have worked collectively for over 12 years to create and share evidence, an approach made possible by relatively stable federal funding. It is unique because it has been able to develop over these years an explicit set of guiding questions, a common theoretical framework and a methodology that draws on multiple disciplines and techniques. It is unique because it understands as decision makers not only those in positions of obvious power, but also women in their various communities. The group has been seeking to share evidence with women in all these communities through a variety of means, some of them innovative in ways that have been copied around the world. It is the combination of approaches that constitutes the claim to uniqueness by Women and Health Care Reform (WHCR, formerly the National Coordinating Group on Women and Health Care Reform), the authors and editors of this book.

This chapter is an introduction both to WHCR and to the book. On the one hand, it is organized chronologically, tracing the development of strategies over the dozen years. On the other hand, the chapter is developed thematically, explaining how the group came to explore particular issues and how those issues are updated here. The chronological and thematic are intertwined, illustrating how projects progress over time and in relation to other developments in health care. The real story, though, is what is happening to our health care system as it undergoes multiple reforms and the consequences of reforms for women as a group and for particular groups of women. To tell that story, we have created individual chapters focused on specific themes while uniting them through our shared approach. At the same time, we wrote the chapters so they could be used independently. As a result, there is occasionally some overlap in material.

## Locating Reform

Throughout the twentieth century, health care in Canada has been punctuated by fundamental change followed by slower adjustment. The 1990s marked the beginning of a new transformative stage, so significant that it was termed "health care reform." The federal government played a major role in this development. Although the Canadian Constitution declares health care to be mainly a provincial and territorial responsibility, the federal government has provided direct services to the military, the RCMP, some First Nations and Inuit peoples, and has also shaped provincial services in direct and indirect ways. Signing international agreements, placing regulations on drugs and immigration, and targeting funding for research and infrastructure are just some of the ways the federal government influences health care in the provinces and territories. The most obvious federal influence is through the 1984 *Canada Health Act*, the legislation that sets out the five principles of accessibility, universality, comprehensiveness, portability, and public administration that the provincial governments are required to meet in order to be eligible for federal funding. The federal funding was significantly reduced in the 1990s, prompting reforms in the provinces and territories.

On a much smaller scale, in 1996 the federal government introduced the Women's Health Contribution Program, which had as its centrepiece five centres of excellence for women's health and the Canadian Women's Health Network (CWHN). These centres were intended to establish a research agenda that asked new questions in new ways about women's health needs and the conditions that shape women's health. Equally important, the centres were intended to be influenced by and influence women in their varied communities. They were a significant part of the federal international commitments to gender equity. That health care reforms were made a major concern by this government program is not surprising, given that women are the majority of both those receiving care and of those providing care, and that dramatic changes were underway. Health care reforms were in the news and the Women's Health Bureau recognized that this was a women's issue.

The National Coordinating Group on Health Care Reform and Women was established in 1997 as part of the Women's Health Contribution Program, with members from each of the centres of excellence and CWHN. (At roughly the same time, the program also funded Women and Health Protection, a group concerned about the safety of pharmaceutical drugs.) The mandate of our group was to coordinate research on health care reform across the centres, to identify and fill gaps, to influence policy, and to share knowledge with a wide variety of women. As was the case with the Women's Health Contribution Program as a whole, our mandate was consistent with Canada's long history of international commitments to equity and with the federal plan to apply a gender-based analysis in all policy development (Clow et al., Ch. 1, 2009).

In the years since then, the centres, the CWHN, and Women and Health Care Reform have refined and further developed this approach, now usually using the term "sex- and gender-based analysis" (SGBA). Based on the work funded by the Women's Health Contribution Program, *Rising to the Challenge: Sex and Gender-Based Analysis for Health Planning, Policy, and Research in Canada* (Clow et al., Ch. 1, 2009) explains in some detail that sex is a term frequently used to identify biological characteristics, while gender usually refers to socially constructed ones. Fausto-Stirling's work (2005, 2006) demonstrates that there is no clear distinction between sex and gender, with our very biology shaped by social relations, but the distinction is useful in emphasizing that we always need to think about bodies, social conditions, and social relations together. Sex- and gender-based analysis has thus become the current way of describing the central goal of the program.

## Establishing a Framework

This book builds on the work of Women and Health Care Reform, taking the 1990s as our starting point. Our task has been daunting, made no less so by the complexity of a system with 14 different jurisdictions and the lack of any single, coordinating organization or other source that documents reforms. Our history is one of first establishing basic principles, then applying these to specific themes. We have sought both to take up current issues and to identify new areas of concern to women. To do so, we have drawn mainly on existing research and applied a gender lens, but we have also produced new data.

4

Our first project was to establish an approach, which we did by identifying three major questions: (1) Why is health care reform a woman's issue? (2) What are the issues for women? and (3) Which women are affected by health care reform? These questions have guided our work throughout our years of research, publishing, policy interventions, and knowledge-sharing at the national, regional, local, and community levels. These questions remain relevant to current issues and provide the guide for this book.

Our second project was to develop a framework for examining the disparate and confusing health care reforms. Over a long weekend we struggled together to develop a shared way of seeing the complex issues involved in health care reforms. Based on our knowledge of developments in health care, on our feminist political economy perspective, and on previous approaches (Armstrong, Armstrong & Connelly, 1997), we came to the conclusion that the reforms could best be understood as versions of privatization. We broadened the common definition of privatization to extend it beyond questions of ownership or delivery and identified what we saw as five main forms that would make the processes of reforms more visible.

One form of privatization we identified was the adoption of for-profit managerial practices in the organization and delivery of services. Hospitals were closed and others amalgamated, imitating corporations and eliminating jobs in the female-dominated workforce. Work was analyzed in terms of discrete tasks, with the data used as the basis for reducing staff to the absolute minimum and for increasing control over the women providing care. Patient stays were shortened and outpatient services expanded, with the result that all those who stayed longer in hospital required intensive and complex care. Casual and part-time work became more common at the same time as the workload increased for those with full-time work.

A second form was the privatization of delivery, with more of the work handed over to for-profit firms. Within the non-profit services, which included almost all hospitals, many long-term care facilities, and home-care operations, work such as cleaning, laundry, cooking, clerical, and management were defined out of what constitutes care and contracted to for-profit firms that had previously primarily serviced hotels and universities. Here, too, the number of employees was reduced and work intensified. Salaries were lowered in the process and benefits disappeared along with job security. Through competitive bidding, which often favoured for-profit firms, whole services such as residential care and cataract surgeries were contracted to for-profit firms.

A third form was the privatization of work. With patients sent home "quicker and sicker," and entry into residential care subject to stricter requirements, more care was left to be done mainly by women at home. These women usually work without pay or formal training and often with little formal support. The privatization of care work is connected to the fourth and fifth forms, the privatization of payment and the privatization of responsibility. The privatization of payment was often invisible until people sought services. More fees were charged for services and some services, such as eye care, were no longer covered by the public health care system or medicare, as it is usually called. This form of privatization is particularly problematic for women because more women than men are poor, and because fewer women than men have their extra health services covered through workplace benefits. The fifth form is about people being expected to take more responsibility for their own health, both before and after treatment. Here, too, it is women who bear the brunt of the privatization because it is women who are expected to keep their families healthy and who are often held responsible for illness understood as preventable. For example, children sent to school with a cold, children who are not washing their hands, children who are not eating their broccoli or exercising are increasingly seen as a personal problem that can be traced to mothers.

# Asking the Questions: Applying the Framework

Using this privatization frame, we commissioned papers intended not only to identify major reforms but also to analyze their impact on women. This work demonstrated that reforms were an issue for women and that the impact varied significantly among women, at the same time as it revealed the paucity of gender-based analysis in the field. Eventually published as a book, *Exposing Privatization* (Armstrong et al., 2002) and as a "plain-language" document or what we called a "popular piece," our initial focus on privatization set a pattern for future work. The popular pieces became models for disseminating knowledge and prompting discussion, with bodies such as the Pan American Health Organization copying our strategy and translating our materials in the same format for their members. At the same time, the book provided an entry point for more academic and policy interventions.

This work on privatization began our exploration of theory and methods, of ways of seeing and of doing research. Chapter 1 in this volume reflects and expands on how our theory-methods framework has developed since then and provides a way forward for the still necessary work on health care reform. *Exposing Privatization* was also the first step in our focus on health care work, a subject that is updated and expanded in the chapters on women's work in health care (Chapter 7), and on the mental health of health care workers (Chapter 8). Moreover, this privatization framework is essential to understanding what is happening in long-term care (Chapter 5), in home care (Chapter 6), and in private health insurance (Chapter 10). Indeed, privatization in all its forms remains a powerful force shaping women's care labour.

Privatization offered both a frame and a basis for exploring health care reforms in general. From there, we moved to concentrate on specific aspects of the system in an effort to shape and respond to new developments in health services in ways that made gender visible. We began by focusing on home care, an issue that was just emerging as critical to reforms. We wanted an approach that would not simply produce more evidence, preach to the converted, or call for more research. We struggled to find an innovative way to follow through on our notion that knowledge could be simultaneously created and shared, could be based on evidence, and both produced in and linked to practice. We settled on a new kind of workshop—or "think garden," as participants relabelled it—that brought together 55 people from the policy, research, and practitioner communities to discuss home care and unpaid work. The participants were selected based on their knowledge of or experience in health services and/or women's issues and policy-making. Commissioned papers on women and home care were distributed before the three-day meeting, providing the soil and fertilizer for moving beyond what has been done to create new knowledge.

The result was magical. You had to be there to experience the collective creation of knowledge. Participants decided that we already knew enough about women, home care, and unpaid care provision to set out principles paralleling those in the *Canada Health Act*. The collective result was *The Charlottetown Declaration on the Right to Care*, included here as Appendix 1, which made clear how women's issues can be integrated into policy in ways that benefit the society as a whole. The *Declaration* was picked up and used by women's health organizations in various parts of the world and stands up today as a guide to establishing equitable health services, especially but not exclusively in home care.

This work on home care also resulted in a book, *Caring for/Caring About*, and a plain-language document, as well as in numerous policy presentations before governments and community organizations. Chapter 6 picks up many of the threads from that research and examines how far we have—or have not—come since then. Home care remains a hot topic, particularly in light of new concerns about an aging population, as Chapter 5 on long-term care makes clear. The two chapters on work—chapters 6 and 7—also take up aspects of unpaid care because it is unpaid workers who provide the majority of care and who featured as central figures in our workshop deliberations. The home care workshop was the first in a long series of workshops organized by WHCR—workshops that were constantly taking new forms and new approaches in an effort to stimulate knowledge and policy creation in areas that had been unexplored through a gender lens.

One issue that was continually emerging in our work was the matter of evidence and, related to that, research methods. Following on the publication of articles on gender-based analysis and methods (Grant, 2000, 2002), we organized a workshop intended to critically examine evidence by framing the issues around indicators. We began by asking who counts and what is counted as evidence in organizing services and in practising care. This questioning resulted in another popular piece, titled *Just the Facts, Ma'am ... A Women's Guide for Understanding Evidence about Health and Health Care* (2005). It was our most difficult popular piece because it challenged us to walk a fine line between academic and popular work, and between demonstrating how all evidence is contingent and how we need evidence as a basis in health service, evidence that pays attention to women as well as to differences among women. We further explored evidence by challenging conventional approaches to investigating wait times, using the specific example of surgery to replace hips and knees to show how simply counting the number of women and men who have surgery fails to determine equity in care (Jackson, Pederson & Boscoe, 2009). Our gender lens then prompted us to fashion a workshop that used wait times to expand the evidence issue, arguing that wait times can only be understood through a gender-based analysis that takes context and inequities into account. This, in turn, led us to question a gold standard in health services research, the systematic review. In our efforts to figure out how to ensure that SGBA is part of the assessment of quality research, we have come to the conclusion that such reviews are about universalizing in ways that remove context. Yet gender analysis, especially when concerned with all forms of equity, makes context central. All of these issues, and more, are taken up in Chapter 1 on theory and methods. The more specific issue of systematic reviews is examined in Chapter 3, which promotes a gender-sensitive approach to assessing evidence.

Just as primary health care was returning to the national agenda, we organized yet another workshop about the issues in primary health care. Challenging the participants from the research, policy, and practitioner communities to *Dare to Dream* (Pederson & Jackson, 2004), based on a discussion paper distributed to participants before the sessions (Pederson & Donner, 2004), our goal was to determine how primary health care services could be designed to meet the needs of women in all their diversity. In this case, as elsewhere in our work, we spent time on the terminology because it has important implications. As Chapter 2 explains, there are significant distinctions between primary care and primary health care. With primary health care once more highlighted in health services planning, it is particularly important to recognize why gender matters and how it matters in such care. Chapter 2 expands on the issues we identified for women in our popular piece on the topic.

Designing long-term residential care with women in mind, the title of a 2007 workshop was an equally difficult task. It is particularly challenging to think about alternatives when the work and care in such facilities is assigned so little value, in part because it is women caring for women. As is the case with health care reforms in general, it is hard to get a handle on what long-term care looks like in Canada. Indeed, it is even harder because this service is not so obviously subject to the principles of the *Canada Health Act*, which encourages at least some uniformity in hospital and doctor care. Again, as in the case of health care reform in general, we had to begin by commissioning work to identify the landscape and provide a background bibliography to create a basis for exchange. *A Place to Call Home* (Armstrong et al., 2009) brought together the presentations from that workshop, supplemented by papers commissioned to fill gaps identified there. The issues for women have become even more urgent as policy debates focus on the assumed threat to the health care system posed by an aging population, threats that are mainly about women, given our longevity, our poverty, and our majority in long-term care. Chapter 5 on long-term care highlights the major themes, while integrating more recent research.

For years, Women and Health Care Reform avoided the health services and topics most often associated with women's health, both because we wanted to emphasize that all issues are women's issues and because more work had been done on those areas. So we focused on neglected areas. However, with what we saw as both major threats and major opportunities in developments in health services related to traditional women's issues, we turned our attention to maternity care. Our popular piece *Maternity Matters* (2007) asked why we should care about the state of maternity care in Canada, highlighting the most significant concerns not only for women but for the system as a whole. As part of a workshop on women's health and maternal environments, we commissioned papers on the care provider environment, examining who is available to provide what kind of care to whom. The issues we raised there are still critical for women today and new ones are emerging, as Chapter 4 in this volume makes clear.

Throughout our history, Women and Health Care Reform has sought to anticipate and promote issues that have not received much attention and have received virtually none from women's perspective. One such issue is quality. Many health reforms have been undertaken in the name of quality, but few have asked women what quality means to them. WHCR did that, and we report our findings in Chapter 9. Private health insurance provides another example. The shift in responsibility for both care and payment has meant more reliance on private health care insurance, at the same time as more employed women have increasingly limited access to such benefits through their paid employment. Our commissioned paper (Jenkins, 2007) on private health insurance demonstrated that such a shift has a differential impact, increasing inequities in access not only between women and men but also among women. This research provided a basis for policy talks at the federal level and for yet another popular piece. We have updated and expanded that analysis in Chapter 10.

In keeping with our practice of constantly moving in new directions, we have identified emerging issues in this book. While each chapter provides current information and indicates new areas for research and action, Chapter 11 takes on an issue we have not addressed before. Obesity has been the focus of health promotion strategies, which is one reason for us to take it on. We, however, seek to apply a somewhat different lens. Chapter 11 aims to establish why obesity is a women's issue, to explore the impact on women, and to look at differences among women. Chapter 12, the final chapter, looks ahead. It identifies areas that require research and many that require action.

This book does not provide a comprehensive landscape of reform. Rather, our purpose is to show why and how gender matters by using specific cases. Such an analysis requires us to talk explicitly about theory, methods, and evidence and to demonstrate the application of these approaches through the exploration of specific aspects of health care reforms. It is intended to share knowledge and prompt both debate and policy action. It is also intended to reflect our collective wisdom. While individuals took primary responsibility for the chapters that bear their names, the material in each builds on our past work together and is the product of a shared assessment.

# References

Armstrong, H., Armstrong, P. & Connelly, M. (1997). The many forms of privatization. *Studies in Political Economy* 53(Summer), 3–9.

Armstrong, P., et al. (2002). *Exposing privatization: Women and health care reform in Canada.* Aurora: Garamond Press.

Armstrong, P., et al. (2009). *A place to call home: Long-term care in Canada.* Halifax: Fernwood.

Clow, B., et al. (2009). *Rising to the challenge: Sex and gender-based analysis for health planning, policy, and research in Canada.* Halifax: Atlantic

Centre of Excellence for Women's Health. Retrieved from http://www.acewh.dal.ca/pdf/Rising_to_the_challenge.pdf

Fausto-Sterling, A. (2005). Bare bones of sex: Part I, sex and gender. *Signs 30*(2), 1491–1527.

Fausto-Sterling, A. (2006). Bare bones of sex: Part II, race and bones. *Social Studies of Science 38*(5), 657–694.

Grant, K. (2000). *Is there a method to this madness? Studying health care as if women mattered.* Prepared for the National Coordinating Group on Health Care Reform and Women. Retrieved from http://www.womenandhealthcarereform.ca/publications/method-madness.pdf

Grant, K. (2002). *GBA: Beyond the red queen syndrome.* Retrieved from http://www.womenandhealthcarereform.ca/en/work_evidence.html

Grant, K., et al. (2004). *Caring for/Caring about: Women, homecare, and unpaid caregiving.* Aurora: Garamond Press.

Jackson, B., Pederson, A. & Boscoe, M. (2009). Waiting to wait: Improving wait time evidence through gender-based analysis. In P. Armstrong & J. Deadman (Eds.), *Women's health intersections of policy, research, and practice* (pp. 35–52). Toronto: Women's Press.

Jenkins, A. (2007). *Women and private health insurance: A review of the issues.* Report Commissioned by Women and Health Care Reform.

Pederson, A. & Donner, L. (2004). *Women and primary health care reform: A discussion paper.* Prepared for the National Workshop on Women and Primary Health Care Winnipeg. Retrieved from http://www.womenandhealthcarereform.ca/en/work_primary.html

Pederson, A. & Jackson, B. (2004). *Dare to dream: Reflections on a national workshop on women and primary health care.* Retrieved from http://www.womenandhealthcarereform.ca/publications/nphcworkshopreport.pdf

Women and Health Care Reform. (2005). *Just the facts, ma'am ... A women's guide for understanding evidence about health and health care.* Retrieved from http://www.womenandhealthcarereform.ca/en/work_evidence.html

Women and Health Care Reform. (2007). *Maternity matters.* http://www.womenandhealthcarereform.ca/en/work_maternity.html Women and Health Care Reform.

CHAPTER 1

# Theory and Methods for Thinking Women

## BETH JACKSON

[W]e are actively committed to struggling against racial, sexual, heterosexual, and class oppression, and see as our particular task the development of integrated analysis and practice based upon the fact that the major systems of oppression are interlocking. The synthesis of these oppressions creates the conditions of our lives.

— *The Combahee River Collective [1977] 1983, 264*

In this chapter, we describe the theoretical and methodological tools that Women and Health Care Reform applies in our research on health care reform, women's health, and health equity. In brief, our "knowledge project" is informed by multidisciplinary feminist approaches to health systems, women's health, and the production of data, evidence, and knowledge in science and policy-making, taking into account the multiple and overlapping contexts in which these data, evidence, and knowledge are produced and circulated.

Our theory and methods form a collective practice that has emerged in an iterative journey over the course of the 13 years that we have worked together. Our process is grounded not only in the theoretical traditions of feminist political economy and feminist approaches to science, it is also informed by the robust yet flexible tools of sex- and gender-based analysis and intersectionality. We have applied these approaches with a keen commitment to documenting the impact of health care reforms on women's lives across a range of social locations. We have focused on processes of change that support equity, and the various contexts in which inequities are produced and transformative acts of social justice occur—that is, in the domains of government policy, institutional structures, and interpersonal practices. In our work, context is critical and women are a credible and important source of knowledge about their experiences and the contexts that shape them.

All of our research is framed around three key, interrelated questions:

1. Why is this a women's issue?
2. What are the issues for women?
3. Which women are affected in what ways? This question takes into account social, economic, and physical locations, and asks what the issues mean for women as patients, providers, and decision-makers, with the understanding that these are frequently overlapping categories.

We recognize that health care reform issues are not only about women; nevertheless, women are our primary concern, given their significant overrepresentation as paid and unpaid care providers. Moreover, we grapple with the tension between "lumping" diverse women together and "splitting" the overall category according to various configurations of identity and social location as we undertake our analysis. In the end, we use the overall category of "women" strategically in our work, at the same time as we recognize the importance of women's different experiences and access to power/resources. We start our analysis with women as a coherent category because, as Beck ([1986] 1992) points out, health care systems and other institutions commonly treat women as a group, and as if they have specific, shared risks—and frequently, the result is shared risks. However, we also understand that the category of women is complex and intersects with many other social locations (e.g., racialization, ethnicity, age, sex, class, sexual orientation, citizenship, status/migration experience, disability)—and systems of power and privilege operate differently across these locations and have different effects. So, while we start with women as a group, our question of "Which women?" shifts our analysis to the multiple, sometimes contradictory social positions that women occupy and the ways in which the benefits and burdens of health care reforms are distributed among women.

Overall, our approach to addressing health care reforms and women

- shifts the health research paradigm away from male-centred or genderless populations or narrowly defined women's problems, to assume that all issues are women's issues; while gender is never the only social location that matters, it matters all the time in both subtle and overt ways;
- expands the categories, showing how single issues are embedded in complex relationships with other issues; policies and practices are deployed at multiple levels, from individual households to global forums;
- challenges reductionist, disease-focused biomedical models and universalizing approaches that homogenize women's experiences;
- emphasizes context, recognizing the specificities of women's lives;
- supports the use of multiple methods and insists on the inclusion of women's voices;
- anticipates new issues, articulating them for women as a group and for particular groups of women;

17

- develops multiple means for sharing the production and
  distribution of research.

In the following sections, we describe in more detail some of the
theoretical and methodological tools that have guided and shaped
our analysis of health care reforms and women.

The theory-methods package we have constructed over the course
of our work is located at the nexus of feminist political economy,
feminist epistemology, sex- and gender-based analysis (SGBA),
and intersectionality. The common themes among the elements
of our framework include: the importance of situating (multiply
positioned) women in practices of production and reproduction;
the necessity of accounting for material conditions (political, economic, social, corporeal) within an advanced and nuanced understanding of the practices and outcomes of power, privilege, and
inequality; and the value of including women's voices and experiences as authoritative and credible sources of knowledge.

## Feminist Political Economy

The political economy refers to the institutions and relations that
comprise political, economic, social, ideological, and cultural
systems (Armstrong & Armstrong, 1996). Political economy perspectives emphasize material relations, social structures, modes
of production ("the ways in which people produce, consume and
allocate the products of human labour" [Luxton & Bezanson,
2006, 24]) and social class, with a particular focus on how a dominant class "by virtue of its control over the means of production,
can compel the labour of another class and appropriate the wealth
produced by the labouring class for its own consumption" (Luxton & Bezanson, 2006, 20).

Within this tradition, feminist political economy is similarly concerned with the material practices of power and the distribution of

social resources. Feminist political economy understands gender and class as interrelated systems of power that work through and are continuously (re)constituted by social relations of production and reproduction. It examines how both gender and class shape social and political relationships and structures, and the differential political and economic effects that flow from these relationships and structures (Inter Pares, 2004). A central contribution of feminist political economy is the concept of "social reproduction," which refers to "the activities and attitudes, behaviours and emotions, responsibilities and relationships, directly involved in the maintenance of life on a daily basis, and intergenerationally" (Laslett & Brenner, cited in Luxton & Bezanson, 2006, 34–35). This includes, but is not limited to, the production, preparation, and/or maintenance of food, clothing, and housing; child care and rearing; elder care; and care of the sick/infirm. "Social reproduction can thus be seen to include various kinds of work—mental, manual, and emotional—aimed at providing the historically, socially, as well as biologically, defined care necessary to maintain existing life and to reproduce the next generation" (Laslett & Brenner, cited in Luxton & Bezanson, 2006, 34–35). The concept of social reproduction demonstrates how both paid employment and unpaid domestic labour are part of the same economic processes "of production and consumption that in combination generate the household's livelihood" (Luxton & Bezanson, 2006, 37). In the end, capitalism as a mode of production *depends on* social reproduction "whether it is achieved through a sex/gender division of labour based on women's unpaid domestic labour and rooted in the heterosexual nuclear family form or, as is true for immigrants, an international division of labour reliant primarily on resources (including women's unpaid domestic labour) from a sending country" (Vosko, 2002, 77).

Three key concerns are addressed by feminist political economy: the sexual division of labour, the role of the state, and the construction and relationship between the public and private spheres (Vosko, 2002). First, the sexual division of labour refers to the assignment of specific forms of work to different sexes, and the differential valuation of those forms of work. Feminist political economy has analyzed the sexual division of labour in key areas such as wage inequality, the sex/gender division of labour in households, and labour market segmentation by sex. It has also located the roots of women's disadvantaged position as waged and unwaged workers. Second, the role of the state refers to "the state's contribution to the reproduction of the [patriarchal capitalist] mode of production" (Jensen, cited in Vosko, 2002, 63). Women and Health Care Reform uses theoretically grounded, applied case studies of health care reforms and their impact on women to examine the role of the state in this reproduction of capitalist systems, and to develop a description of how that role is organized. Third, feminist political economy pays close attention to the role that the public and private spheres play in gendered relations of production and reproduction. The public sphere is generally associated with politics, government, markets, and workplaces, and the private sphere is associated with the so-called natural domestic elements of social life (e.g., family, sexuality, child/elder care). Feminist political economy examines the construction of these spheres and how they reinforce and recreate one another.

Despite its contributions, feminist political economy has been subject to the same critique as its more mainstream counterparts—that it has privileged economic relations over others, thus failing to recognize how race, ethnicity, and other social locations have shaped class relations. Creese and Stasiulis (1996) have urged a fundamental rethinking of political economy: "The intersection of multiple axes of power and meaning must become as central to understanding the material world, the organization of local and global economies, national and transnational state systems, as they are, in complex and often contradictory ways, to our individual and collective experience of the world, and our efforts to change it" (Creese & Stasiulis, 1996, 9). Over the past two decades, feminist scholarship in political economy has begun to explore, more deeply than ever before, how the interrelationships among class, gender, race, and ethnicity shape women's relationship to capitalism (Vosko, 2002). Inspired by a broad range of feminist theorizing, feminist political economy is now invested in exploring the multiple intersections of gender, race, and class (as well as other social locations) and the complex power relationships enacted through them.

## Feminist Epistemologies

Feminist epistemologies (theories of how we know things) inspire us to provide responsible accounts of how and what we know, and to locate those accounts in their social, political, and historical contexts. A crucial part of this is articulating the assumptions upon which knowledge claims are based. Broadly speaking, mainstream science is based on several "objectivist-realist" epistemological foundations, which are countered by feminist "materialist" epistemologies:

1. Mainstream science is based on a "correspondence" theory of truth that assumes that we can know things through direct experience or through instruments of observation, and that what our senses can perceive corresponds to what is real. This assumes that objects of knowledge are finite, stable, unified (internally coherent and whole in themselves), and independent of the existence of knowers (i.e., not shaped in any way by how we do/do not perceive them or by the methods we use to perceive them).

2. Feminist epistemologies take a more "constructivist" view of truth and evidence, asserting that our perceptions are always a function of not only our methods of observation but our physical embodiment and social location in complex relations of power.

3. Mainstream, objectivist science embraces "epistemological individualism," the view that knowledge is the

outcome of an individual activity in which a knower grasps truths that are independent of the contexts in which they are understood.

4. Nelson (1990) and other feminist epistemologists claim that this approach is implausible, arguing that individuals' knowledge activities occur in the context of communities that construct and share knowledge and standards of evidence. In other words, there are no dislocated truths and no dislocated knowers—research and knowledge are granted authority and legitimated by communities. Evidence "speaks in a discursive space that is made available, prepared for it" (Code, 1995, 43; see also Longino, 1992).

5. Mainstream science holds that all human subjects share universal qualities that make them essentially interchangeable as knowers. To the extent that mainstream science acknowledges human differences, the conventional view is that this diversity can be contained by strict standards and rules for scientific inquiry. In other words, an objectivist approach to science and knowledge assumes it is possible to bracket any particularity that might intrude upon an individual's neutral observation. Consequently, any human subject can be an impartial observer.

This attitude treats the gender, race, class, sexuality, and other social locations of knowers as inconsequential. But to dismiss these differences "as though they simply constitute differences in situations in which one finds oneself—is to underappreciate the depth at which such structures operate in our lives" (Scheman, 1995, 178, cited in Tuana, 2001, 4). Feminist approaches to knowledge deem it inconceivable that our experiences in structured relations of power (e.g., race, class, gender) have no bearing on the type of knowledge we pursue or create. Acknowledging the impact of these social locations on our knowledge practices is an important step toward taking responsibility for the knowledge we produce and circulate (Code, 1995). Moreover, feminist epistemologists assert that objectivist epistemologies mistakenly ignore embodiment, a critical aspect of subjectivity and an important context for knowledge production. Nancy Tuana explains: "The model of the generic knower has traditionally ignored or minimized the epistemic relevance of our bodily differences. Attention to the body calls attention to the specificities and partiality of human knowledge, as well as reminding us of the importance of acknowledging the role of materiality [...] in the knowledge process" (Tuana, 2001, 9). The affirmation of both social location and physical embodiment as crucial elements in knowledge production distinguishes a feminist "material-discursive" epistemology from the "objectivist-realist" epistemology that underpins much mainstream science.

In sum, a feminist material-discursive epistemology acknowledges that knowers, objects of knowledge, and knowledge practices (e.g., measurement and analysis) exist always and only in specific contexts, and that what we observe and know is grounded both in social meanings and practices (culture) and in material reality (nature). In other words, our measurements and observations are not simply a mirror of "what is," nor are they simply discursive (cultural products) — rather, our observations and evidence are always grounded both in systems of discourse and in material reality. While there is no essential truth to be discovered, neither is our experience of the world insubstantial or entirely relative; the world pushes back against us, resisting attempts to say "anything goes." (*Warning:* Don't try to walk through a wall, or breach a social norm without consequence.) So our best efforts at knowledge production are those that account for the specific conditions in and locations from which we experience, observe, and interpret reality. Donna Haraway (1991, 195) tells us that this is an epistemology "of location, positioning, and situating, where partiality and not universality is the condition of being heard to make rational knowledge claims. These are claims on people's lives; the

23

view from a body, always a complex, contradictory, structuring and structured body, versus the view from above, from nowhere, from simplicity." For our evidence to be responsible, we must account for the material conditions, the social contexts, and the instruments of observation for the knowledge claims we make.

# Sex- and Gender-Based Analysis

> Sex- and gender-based analysis (SGBA) investigates known or potential implications for women, men, boys and girls by examining physiological and social phenomena, including processes that organize social relations, generate identities and structure social institutions. (Adapted from Johnson, Greaves & Repta, 2007)

Sex and gender are closely associated but distinct concepts. The term "sex" is used to describe biological, anatomical, and physiological aspects (e.g., skeletal and reproductive structures, hormones) of humans and other animals (Johnson, Greaves & Repta, 2007). "Gender" is a term that is applied almost exclusively to humans; is culturally specific and temporal; and refers to the social roles, meanings, and status that are applied to people in different sex categories. It affects the distribution of social, political, and economic power and resources and, consequently, opportunities for health, household and relationship experiences, and for community engagement. While it has often been understood that sex and gender map neatly onto one another—humans of the male sex have masculine characteristics and occupy social positions as men, while humans of the female sex have feminine characteristics and occupy social positions as women—the binary categories implied by these terms have been challenged by recent social theory and social movements that have broadened our understanding of sex and gender to include intersex, transgender, and other culturally specific sex/gender categories. In other words, there is no simple dichotomy between sex and gender, between bodies and their social and physical environments—while they are discrete concepts, they are also fluid and interactive. Moreover, there are significant physiological differences among women and among men, as well as differences between women and men in how their bodies are interpreted and experienced. To complicate matters further, sex and gender also affect health through their interaction with other social locations and key determinants of health, including income, paid and unpaid work, age, disability, racialization, geography, migration experience, and language. These interactions of sex and gender with other social relations and locations produce health advantages and inequities. While increasingly sophisticated accounts of sex and gender have gained ground in health research in recent years (Annandale, 2009) and have helped to spur research in important directions, it remains difficult to disentangle these multiple biological and social factors to measure their effects on health, access to and provision of health services, and experiences in health systems.

Nevertheless, understanding how sex and gender affect health and health care remains an important task because both sex and gender affect trajectories, prevalence, and treatment of health conditions and diseases. In Canada, as elsewhere in the world, there are significant sex and gender differences in health and health-related inequities.[1] For example, on average, women live longer than men, but women die prematurely more often than men from largely preventable conditions such as cervical cancer and lung cancer; die in the prime of life more often than men because of sex-specific conditions (e.g., breast cancer versus prostate cancer); and experience higher levels of disability than men, especially in their later years (Morrow, Hankivsky & Varcoe, 2007).

In Canada, sex- and gender-based analysis has a long history (beyond the scope of this chapter) that is grounded in the women's health movement and is supported by numerous policy commitments at all levels of government (Morrow et al., 2007; Reid et al., 2007; Tudiver, 2009).[2] The conduct of SGBA has been the subject of several primers, guides, and case-study publications (e.g., Benoit & Shumka, 2009; Clow et al., 2009; Hankivsky & Cormier, 2009; Johnson et al., 2007; Spitzer et al., 2007), and the rest of the chapters in this book document the application of SGBA to health care reforms and their impact on women. In general, sex- and gender-based analyses pose and strive to answer core, sensitizing questions that mirror the questions outlined at the beginning of this chapter. While Women and Health Care Reform has chosen to focus our analysis on women, this work is embedded in the broader questions implied by a sex- and gender-based analysis: What is the distribution of power and resources among differently sexed and gendered groups? What is the distribution of effects/outcomes? What are the pathways (at micro [individual], meso [e.g., institutional or community], and macro [societal] levels) through which these effects occur? Who benefits and who bears the costs? In sum, sex- and gender-based analysis

- attends to social, historical, and political contexts of gendered social relations;
- draws upon multiple research methods and forms of data and evidence (e.g., randomized clinical trials, population-level survey data, health impact assessments, systematic reviews, and narrative and arts-based methods and data);
- is an iterative process of critical thinking, not a formulaic checklist;
- critically assesses implications of policies and programs by assembling data and assessing gaps, looking for intended and unintended consequences, describing context, and identifying blind spots.

A robust sex- and gender-based analysis is complemented by an intersectional approach, which has a unique history and focuses on the complex intersections and influences of multiple social locations.

# Intersectionality

> Intersectional theory argues that gender, race, ethnicity, sexuality, and class are mutually constitutive, intersect in the lived experiences of those who occupy and negotiate different social locations in systems of power in the health care system and in the larger society, and that health inequalities are produced by racism, gender inequality, and class relations. (Weber & Fore, 2007)

In 1977, the Combahee River Collective, a group of Black lesbian feminists in Boston, published the historic statement on their politics and work—including the concept of interlocking systems of oppression—that opens this chapter. The term "intersectionality" was later coined by legal scholar Kimberlé Crenshaw (1989) to describe the tangled connections between gender and race, sexism and racism, and how they interact to shape the multiple dimensions of Black women's experiences. Over the last two decades, intersectionality has been further developed as an interdisciplinary approach to understanding the operation and effects of multiple systems of social relations and hierarchy (e.g., gender, racialization, class, and sexuality) (Hankivsky & Cormier, 2009; Weber & Parra-Medina, 2003; Weber & Fore, 2007). Intersectionality takes the position that "social identities which serve as organizing features of social relations, mutually constitute, reinforce, and naturalize one another" (Shields 2008, 302).[3] That is, the boundaries, meaning, experiences, and material effects associated with one category (e.g., gender) are created and maintained in continuous and dynamic interaction with the boundaries, meaning, experiences, and material effects associated with other categories (e.g., age, race, class). Moreover, there are important *relational* and *contradictory* aspects of the intersections of systems of power and structures of domination [whereby] systems of racial, class, gender and sexual domination do not have identical effects on socially constructed categories of

27

women and men" (Creese & Stasiulis, 1996, 8). In other words, while in general men may have more social power than women by virtue of their gender, low-income men or racialized men may, in various circumstances, have less social power than high-income women or White women.

The intersection of identities is not only an individual experience that involves individual engagement, it is a social process that involves the activity of entrenched social discourses (i.e., sets of ideas, beliefs, and practices that both enable and constrain what we can do and know). Intersectionality helps us identify and understand the multiple dimensions of social inequality that manifest at both the macro level of social structures and institutions, and at the micro level of individual experience. At these different levels of social relations, individual and institutional actions, policies, ideologies, and practices work in concert to create disadvantage and privilege through "hierarchies of differential access to a variety of resources—economic, political and cultural" (Yuval-Davis, 2009, 50–51).

Intersectionality is defined not by a single, unified theory or set of methods, but by a core set of sensitizing questions (Weber & Parra-Medina, 2003):

**1. What is the meaning of gender, race, ethnicity, class, sexuality, and other systems of inequality across political and economic domains, institutional structures and individual lives?**

Intersectional analysis bridges macro social structures and embodied experience, contending that interrelated systems at the macro institutional level are created, maintained, and transformed simultaneously and in relationship to one another, while at the micro level of the individual, these systems shape our identities, value systems, perspectives, and interpersonal relations (Weber & Parra-Medina, 2003, 199). The co-creation of these systems and identities occurs in specific historical, political, and geographical contexts and produces distinct social formations. Accounting for context is crucial in our understanding of how intersecting social locations are manifested.

## 2. How are these intersecting systems of inequality produced, reinforced, resisted, and transformed over time, in different social locations, and in different institutional domains?

This question is linked to the first, in that systems of social hierarchy are understood to have "organizational, intersubjective, experiential and representational forms [e.g., images or texts]" (Yuval-Davis, 2009, 49). They are expressed in specific institutions and organizations, such as laws, government agencies, trade unions, voluntary organizations, and families, and they are expressed in everyday interpersonal relationships among people "acting informally and/or in their roles as agents of specific social institutions and structures" (Yuval-Davis, 2009, 49). These systems are human products—they are built, maintained, and transformed by human action. Accordingly, it is important to examine the actions and processes by which they are created, supported, and resisted. Weber (2006, 673) notes: "recognizing that power relations are a central dynamic in race, class, and gender structures is not the same as demonstrating how power relations are co-constructed, maintained, and challenged. And explicating how these systems operate—the mechanisms that constitute and connect them—is a critical challenge before feminist and other scholars."

## 3. How can our understanding of the intersecting dynamics of these systems guide us in the pursuit of social justice?

The pursuit of social justice is a core principle of intersectional theorizing, research, and action. Interventions informed by intersectionality are designed to change macro systems (e.g., economy, education, law) rather than simply focus on altering individual behaviour. When applied to the domain of health, intersectionality can provide a productive alternative to traditional biomedical approaches. Intersectional health scholarship "argues for an expanded conception of health that incorporates a broad framework of social relations and institutions, not just diseases and disorders, and situates health in communities and families, not simply in individual bodies." It "emphasizes power relationships, not just distributional differences in resources, as central to social inequality and health disparities" (Weber & Parra-Medina, 2003, 185). Combined with the insights of feminist political economy, feminist epistemologies, and sex- and gender-based analysis, intersectionality provides a firm footing for investigating the impact of health care reforms on women across a range of social locations.

## Conclusion

The theoretical and methodological instruments we have assembled to address the practices and outcomes of health care reforms provide us with robust tools for our task. Each addresses unique but overlapping concerns. Feminist political economy asks: How are gender, class, and other social locations implicated in political and economic structures, the material practices of power, and the distribution of social resources? It focuses centrally on the sexual division of labour; the role of the state in the reproduction of capitalist systems; the co-construction of the public and private spheres; and how the interrelationships among class, gender, race, and ethnicity shape women's relationship to capitalism.

Feminist epistemologies ask: How do we make responsible knowledge claims about women? In answering, a feminist epistemological approach affirms that both social location (in epistemological communities and socio-political contexts) and physical embodiment (which is assigned meaning in socio-political contexts) are crucial elements in knowledge production. We are reminded that assigning authority to dislocated knowers whose social location and particular characteristics are presumed to have no bearing on what knowledge is sought or produced excuses them from responsibility for the knowledge they create (Code, 1995), and that our best efforts at responsible knowledge production are those that account for the specific conditions in and locations from which we participate in and interpret reality.

Sex- and gender-based analysis asks: What is the distribution of power and resources among differently sexed and gendered groups? How are the outcomes, good and bad, distributed? What are the pathways (at micro, meso, and macro levels) through which these outcomes occur? Who benefits and who bears the costs? In this analysis, social, historical, and political contexts are key, and knowledge is produced through multiple research methods and forms of data and evidence.

And finally, intersectionality asks: What is the meaning of gender, race, ethnicity, class, sexuality, and other systems of inequality across political and economic domains, institutional structures, and individual lives? And how are these intersecting systems of inequality produced, reinforced, resisted, and transformed over time, in different social locations, and in different institutional domains? Some of the earliest formulators of an intersectional analysis, the Combahee River Collective, asserted not only that systems of hierarchy and oppression are interlocking, but that "the synthesis of these oppressions creates the conditions of our lives" (Combahee River Collective, [1977] 1983, p. 264). These systems are not simply ideological, existing only in the realm of thought and political debate—they have important material effects on all of our lives. Michelle Fine entreats us: "While there is a story to be told about each thread, it is the braided story of ideological, material, social and psychological oppression and resistance that must be told. Gender moves across this geography of injustice [...] in dynamic interaction with race, ethnicity, class, and political life" (Guidroz & Berger, 2009, 63).

Thus we have returned to the core questions that define both the origin and destination of our research, and familiar signposts mark the routes of our investigations: the discourses that frame our questions and answers; practices of power, resistance, and resilience; and the material effects of that framing and those practices. Lighting the way are the voices of multiply positioned women, who offer their authoritative and credible accounts of the experiences, relationships, and systems that constitute health care policy, practice, and reform.

# Notes

1. Whitehead and Dahlgren (2006, 2) note that: "Three distinguishing features, when combined, turn mere variations or differences in health into a social inequity in health. They are systematic, socially produced (and therefore modifiable) and unfair."
2. In April 2009, the federal commitment to SGBA in health was reaffirmed by the Health Portfolio (which includes Assisted Human Reproduction Canada, the Canadian Institutes of Health Research, the Hazardous Materials Information Review Commission, Health Canada, the Patented Medicine Prices Review Board, and the Public Health Agency of Canada). This policy commits Government of Canada Health Portfolio members "to use sex and gender-based analysis (SGBA) to develop, implement and evaluate the Health Portfolio's research, programs and policies to address the different needs of men and women, boys and girls." http://www.hc-sc.gc.ca/hl-vs/pubs/women-femmes/sgba-policy-politique-ags-eng.php
3. For example, consider widely accepted North American beliefs about the binary categories of sex (female/male) and gender (women/men) and the many practices related to the reproduction and enforcement of these beliefs and categories. The result of these sex/gender discourses is that categories of male and female are broadly understood as "natural," mapping directly onto the categories of "men" and "women," and denying other possibilities such as multiple, temporary, or fluid genders (Shields, 2008). Luft (2009, 107) notes: "The tireless efforts of sociobiologists to find new biological origins for gendered behaviour, the popular self-help

publications printed every year that assure women and men that a return to their 'natural' roles will bring happiness and successful heterosexual relationships, and the market's insistent reproduction of occupational segregation attest to an ongoing popular obsession with essential gender difference and its 'natural' manifestations."

# References

Annandale, E. (2009). *Women's health and social change.* London: Routledge.

Armstrong, P. & Armstrong, H. (1996). *Wasting away: The undermining of Canadian health care.* Oxford: Oxford University Press.

Beck, U. [1986] (1992). *Risk society, towards a new modernity.* Trans. from the German by Mark Ritter, and with an Introduction by Scott Lash & Brian Wynne. London: Sage Publications.

Benoit, C. & Shumka, L. (2009). *Gendering the health determinants framework: Why girls' and women's health matters.* Vancouver: Women's Health Research Network.

Clow, B., Pederson, A., Haworth-Brockman, M. & Bernier, J. (Eds.). (2009). *Rising to the challenge: Sex- and gender-based analysis for health planning, policy, and research in Canada.* Halifax: Atlantic Centre of Excellence for Women's Health.

Code, L. (1995). *Rhetorical spaces: Essays on gendered locations.* New York: Routledge.

The Combahee River Collective. [1977] (1983). The Combahee River Collective statement. In B. Smith (Ed.), *Home girls, a Black feminist anthology* (pp. 264–274). New York: Kitchen Table Women of Color Press, Inc.

Creese, G. & Stasiulis, D. (1996). Introduction: Intersections of gender, race, class, and sexuality. *Studies in Political Economy* 51(Fall), 5–14.

Crenshaw, K. (1989). Demarginalizing the intersection of race and sex: A Black feminist critique of antidiscrimination doctrine, feminist theory, and antiracist politics. *University of Chicago Legal Forum,* 138–67. Volume 139, pp. 139–167.

Greaves, L. (2009). Women, gender, and health research. In P. Armstrong

& J. Deadman (Eds.), *Women's health: Intersections of policy, research, and practice* (pp. 3–20). Toronto: Women's Press.

Guidroz, K. & Berger, M.T. (2009). A conversation with founding scholars of intersectionality: Kimberlé Crenshaw, Nira Yuval-Davis, and Michelle Fine. In M.T. Berger & K. Guidroz (Eds.), *The intersectional approach: Transforming the academy through race, class, and gender* (pp. 61–80). Chapel Hill: The University of North Carolina Press.

Hankivsky, O. & Cormier, R. (2009). *Intersectionality: Moving women's health research and policy forward.* Vancouver: Women's Health Research Network.

Haraway, D. (1991). *Simians, cyborgs, and women: The reinvention of nature.* New York: Routledge.

Inter Pares. (2004). *Towards a feminist political economy.* Inter Pares Occasional Paper, no. 5 (November). Ottawa. Retrieved from: www.interpares.ca

Jackson, B.E., Pederson, A. & Boscoe, M. (2006). Waiting to wait: Improving wait times evidence through gender-based analysis. In P. Armstrong& J. Deadman (Eds.), *Women's health: Intersections of policy, research, and practice* (pp. 35–51). Toronto: Women's Press.

Johnson, J.L., Greaves, L. & Repta, R. (2007). *Better science with sex and gender: A primer for health research.* Vancouver: Women's Health Research Network.

Longino, H. (1992). Essential tensions—Phase two: Feminist, philosophical, and social studies of science. In E. McMullin (Ed.), *The social dimensions of science* (pp. 198–216). Notre Dame: University of Notre Dame Press.

Luft, R.E. (2009). Intersectionality and the risk of flattening difference: Gender and race logics, and the strategic use of antiracist singularity. In M.T. Berger & K. Guidroz (Eds.), *The intersectional approach: Transforming the academy through race, class, and gender* (pp. 100–117). Chapel Hill: University of North Carolina Press.

Luxton, M. & Bezanson, K. (2006). Feminist political economy in Canada and the politics of social reproduction. In K. Bezanson & M. Luxton (Eds.), *Social reproduction: Feminist political economy challenges neoliberalism* (pp. 11–44). Montreal: McGill-Queen's University Press.

Luxton, M. & Vosko, L. (1998). Where women's efforts count: The 1996 census campaign and "family politics" in Canada. *Studies in Political Economy 56*(Summer), 49–81.

Morrow, M., Hankivsky, O. & Varcoe, C. (Eds.). (2007). *Women's health in Canada: Critical perspectives on theory and policy.* Toronto: University of Toronto Press.

Nelson, L.H. (1990). Epistemological communities. In L. Alcoff & E. Potter (Eds.), *Feminist epistemologies* (pp. 121–160). New York: Routledge.

Popay, J. (Ed.). (2006) *Moving beyond effectiveness in evidence synthesis: Methodological issues in the synthesis of diverse sources of evidence.* National Institute for Health and Clinical Excellence. Retrieved from www.publichealth.nice.org.uk

Reid, C., Pederson, A. & Dupéré, S. (2007). Addressing diversity in health promotion: Implications of women's health and intersectional theory. In M. O'Neill, A. Pederson, S. Dupéré & I. Rootman (Eds.), *Health promotion in Canada: Critical perspectives* (pp. 75–89). Toronto: Canadian Scholars' Press Inc.

Shields, S.A. (2008). Gender: An intersectionality perspective, *Sex Roles 59*, 301–311. DOI 10.1007/s11199-008-9501-8

Spitzer, D.L. & the Gender and Sex-Based Analysis Advisory Committee, Canadian Institutes of Health Research. (2007). *Gender and sex-based analysis in health research: A guide for CIHR peer review committees.* Retrieved from www.cihr-irsc.gc.ca/e/32019.html

Tuana, N. (2001). Material locations: An interactionist alternative to realism/social constructivism. In N. Tuana & S. Morgen (Eds.), *Engendering rationalities* (pp. 221–244). Albany: State University of New York Press.

Tudiver, S. (2009). Integrating women's health and gender analysis in a government context: Reflections on a work in progress. In P. Armstrong & J. Deadman (Eds.), *Women's health: Intersections of policy, research, and practice* (pp. 21–34). Toronto: Women's Press.

Vosko, L. (2002). The pasts (and futures) of feminist political economy in Canada: Reviving the debate. *Studies in Political Economy 68*(Summer), 55–83.

Weber, L. (2006). Reconstructing the landscape of health disparities research. In A.J. Schulz & L. Mullings (Eds.), *Gender, race, class, and health: Intersectional approaches* (pp. 21–59). San Francisco: Jossey-Bass.

Weber, L. & Fore, E. (2007). Race, ethnicity, and health: An intersectional approach. *Handbook of the sociology of racial and ethnic relations*. Retrieved from http://www.cas.sc.edu/wost/images/weber-race.pdf

Weber, L. & Parra-Medina, D. (2003). Intersectionality and women's health: Charting a path to eliminating health disparities. In M.T. Segal, V. Demos & J.J. Kronenfeld (Eds.), *Advances in gender research: Gendered perspectives on health and medicine* (pp. 181–230). Vol. 7(A). San Diego: Elsevier.

Whitehead, M. & Dahlgren, G. (2006). Levelling up (Part 1): A discussion paper on concepts and principles for tackling social inequities in health. *Studies on Social and Economic Determinants of Population Health*, no. 2. WHO Collaborating Centre for Policy Research on Social Determinants of Health, University of Liverpool. Retrieved from https://www.who.int/social_determinants/resources/leveling_up_part1.pdf

Yuval-Davis, N. (2009). Intersectionality and feminist politics. In M.T. Berger & K. Guidroz (Eds.), *The intersectional approach: Transforming the academy through race, class, and gender* (pp. 25–43). Chapel Hill: University of North Carolina Press.

CHAPTER 2

# Primary Health Care for Women in Canada

ANN PEDERSON AND ANNA LIWANDER

## Introduction

Primary care has been described as the "heart of all high-performing health systems" (Webster, 2010, E188) and the foundation of the Canadian health care system. It represents the first point of contact with the health care system for patients and encompasses a wide range of services, including visits to general practitioners, community health centres, or neighbourhood walk-in clinics, calling a provincial health information telephone line, or asking questions of a local pharmacist. Obtaining primary care may mean seeing the same person for care regularly or it can involve visiting a clinic where a variety of practitioners—nurses, doctors, nutritionists, physiotherapists, social workers, midwives—collaborate to provide a comprehensive range of services. Despite the various forms that primary care may take in Canada today, the dominant model of care is that of a physician in a solo or group practice providing care for an established group of patients.

Primary care was one of two areas of health services funded

publicly when "medicare" was established in the 1960s in Canada, the other area being hospital-based care. Most primary care is funded by public insurance programs administered by the 10 provinces and three territories, some of which still charge premiums while others pay for the insurance through various tax programs (Hutchison, Abelson & Lavis, 2001). Core hospital services, on the other hand, are generally free to patients at the point of service and paid for through a variety of operating grants to health authorities and/or hospitals (Armstrong & Armstrong, 2008).

Primary care became an important aspect of contemporary health care reform with the release of *Building on Values: The Future of Health Care in Canada* by the Royal Commission on the Future of Health Care in Canada in late 2002. Led by Roy Romanow, former premier of the province of Saskatchewan and an advocate for publicly funded health care, the report identified "primary health care and prevention" as one of several priorities for action (Romanow, 2002). In so doing, the report entered into a debate over terminology as well as over the changes deemed necessary to improve primary care in Canada.

The debate over terminology centres on the overlapping definitions and parameters of primary care and the closely related but broader concept of primary *health* care introduced by the World Health Organization (WHO) at the international conference on primary health care in Alma Ata, Russia, in 1978 (World Health Organization, n.d.). The two terms—"primary care" and "primary health care"—are understood to denote not only *what* care is delivered in a given health system but also to connote *how, where,* and *by whom.* For many years, primary care in Canada focused on care for acute, episodic problems and/or minor emergencies that could be dealt with outside of hospital. Recent innovations in Canada, however, have begun to confuse the two terms, as new practitioners are granted the right to offer care, new settings are established (such as walk-in clinics without established patient rosters), and the nature of care shifts due to changing illness patterns, demographics, technology, patient demand, and government fiat

(Health Canada, n.d.-b). Today, the traditional reach of primary care is also extending into health promotion, disease prevention, and the management of chronic conditions–precisely the domain of what has been known as primary health care. Increasingly, primary care reforms include advocating for a broader range of services, expanding the types of providers involved (Health Canada, n.d.-b), and shifting the location to include a wide range of facilities, including private offices, community health centres, and clinics on the premises of community-based organizations (Van-Soeren, Hurlock-Chorostecki, Pogue & Sanders, 2008).

Women's health advocates and others have been careful to maintain the historic distinction between primary care and primary health care because the latter concept is based upon a set of values, principles, and practices that are fundamentally different from those directing physician-centred medical services (Donner & Pederson, 2004; Hills & Mullett, 2005; Pederson & Donner, 2007; VanSoeren et al., 2008). Primary health care, as per the Alma Ata Declaration (World Health Organization, n.d.), aligns with many of the aims of women's health reformers, particularly with respect to its understanding and treatment of pregnancy and birth as parts of everyday life and not medical events, and its inclusion of health promotion and disease prevention (including screening and vaccination) as core aspects of care. Moreover, the Alma Ata Declaration names primary health care as a right, challenges governments to address health inequities within and between countries, and recognizes the link between health status and social conditions. It calls for the active involvement of individuals and communities in the design and governance of health care services. For these reasons, many women's health advocates have argued that primary health care provides a good model for meeting women's health care needs in both developed and developing countries (e.g., Hills & Mullett, 2005). In fact, women's health advocates (Hills & Mullett, 2005; Pederson & Donner, 2007; Thurston & O'Connor, 1996) have long called for a primary *health* care system in Canada that includes attention to the social determinants of health, such as income, age, race, and gender, in the design and delivery of health care. The WHO primary health care approach has a greater likelihood of addressing some of the underlying factors that influence women's health status and influence their access to care, ability to provide care, and the outcomes of care. Many women's health advocates have aligned themselves with the international community, calling for primary health care as the backbone of all health care systems (World Health Organization, 2008) and the incorporation of a focus on the determinants of health rather than the narrower focus on health services usually performed by professionals (Rasanathan, Montesinos, Matheson, Etienne & Evans, 2010). As Hills and Mullett (2005) argue, the barriers that women experience in accessing health care are often linked to the social determinants of health and these barriers are often greater for women than for men. This understanding should be integrated into the planning and delivery of primary care.

The interchangeable use of the terms "primary care" and "primary health care" makes reading both the academic and policy literature in this area challenging. However, Australian academic and activist Helen Keleher (2001) has argued that it is important to continue to distinguish between the two terms because of their different practical and political significance in discussions of health reform. In fact, she warns that:

> A slippage in language is counter-productive, first because it disguises the transformative potential of strategies and approaches that can make the fundamental changes necessary to improve health status, and second because the structures and practices of the primary care sector are not necessarily compatible with notions of comprehensive primary health care. There is much to be lost if primary health care and health promotion are disguised as primary care, and not understood for their capacity to make a difference to health inequities although of course in some circumstances,

comprehensive primary health care is interdependent with
services provided by primary care. (Keleher, 2001, 57)

Conscious of this debate, we make an effort to use the terms
"primary care" and "primary health care" as distinct concepts.

In this chapter, we briefly review the nature of primary care
reforms in Canada in the past decade, paying particular attention to initiatives that have occurred since the Romanow Commission and that were supported by $800 million in federal
funding through the Primary Health Care Transition Fund, a
major mechanism for advancing primary care reform from 2000
to 2006 (Health Canada, 2007c). We specifically discuss developments in collaborative care, patient-centred care, and the prevention and management of chronic conditions,[1] areas that have
important implications for women as both providers and receivers of care. We conclude with a discussion of the work of Women
and Health Care Reform, a multidisciplinary group investigating "the effects of health care reforms on women as providers,
decision makers and users of health care systems" (Women and
Health Care Reform, n.d.), and the value of exploring models of
women-centred care.

# Background

Hutchison et al. (2001) argue that primary health care reform in
Canada has been constrained by policy decisions that have led
to a health care system dominated by hospitals, specialists, and
physician-centred primary care. Increasingly, however, patients,
providers, researchers, and governments have questioned
whether a system built primarily to deal with acute episodic
care needs can handle the challenges of providing care for an
aging population with an increasing proportion of chronic conditions. Additionally, concerns have also been raised about the
concentration of health facilities in urban centres and the need

to recognize the distinct health challenges facing rural and First Nations communities (Health Council of Canada, 2010; Hutchison et al., 2001; Ipsos Reid, 2010). In 2000, the first ministers of Canada—the prime minister and provincial and territorial premiers—agreed on a vision of health care renewal that included enhancing access to primary health care (Health Canada, n.d.-a). The Health Accord, due to expire in 2014, set out an action plan with the aim of ensuring "timely access to quality health care on the basis of need and not ability to pay" (Health Canada, n.d.-a). This was supported through funding to improve primary health care, home care, and catastrophic drug coverage, and to support the development of diagnostic and medical equipment, as well as information technology (Health Canada, n.d.-a).

Subsequently, the federal government sponsored a set of innovations and demonstration projects in primary care delivery over six years through the Primary Health Care Transition Fund (PHCTF) (Weatherill, 2007). The prominent areas of focus for these initiatives were collaborative care, chronic disease prevention and management, information management and technology, and evaluation and evidence (Health Canada, 2007c). Since the completion of the PHCTF in 2006, the federal government has played a smaller role in primary care reform, but provincial and territorial governments have continued to act assertively to renew primary care (Hutchison, 2008). Few of the primary health care initiatives supported by the PHCTF concentrated specifically on gender or women's health, except for those that focused on enhancements to maternity care, although innovations in many areas are relevant to women's health (see Health Canada, 2007c).

To date, the major approach to primary care reform in Canada has been to find ways to enhance access to care rather than to address the determinants of health or build linkages between health and other social services (although Quebec has had a different model of care delivery for decades). More specifically, given the organizing and funding principles of the *Canada Health*

*Act,* primary care reform has focused on increasing access to services by increasing the supply of family physicians and general practitioners and/or by increasing access to services through changes in the organization, location, and funding of care. Other approaches have involved using incentives to increase the number of medical students taking up family practice, support for increased enrolments in medical training, and introducing various programs to support family physicians (including new organizational forms of practice, strategies for better communication with other health care providers, and adopting electronic health records and other forms of electronic technology) (Barer, 2002; Beaulieu et al, 2008; Health Canada, n.d.-b; Watson & McGrail, 2009). However, these initiatives have meant only minimal change to the system as a whole and not solved the core problems of having appropriate care available when and where it is needed (Hutchison, 2008). Moreover, physician shortages are not only about the absolute number of physicians available but about where physician resources are deployed (Evans & McGrail, 2008). Thus, physicians are concentrated in urban areas and in some specialty areas rather than necessarily where services are most needed.

This pattern of reforms in primary care is not surprising as it maintains the fundamental commitments enshrined in the *Canada Health Act* and sustains a system of care that enjoys a high level of public support. However, among the emerging directions in primary care reform are initiatives involving *collaborative care (which involves changes in provider mix), patient-centred care,* and *chronic condition prevention and management.* Though this is not an exhaustive list of changes being experimented with in primary care within Canada, these three directions each provide some hope of improved care for all users of primary care, but especially for women, who represent both the main users and providers of health care, including primary care (Pederson & Donner, 2007; Weisman, Chuang & Scholle, 2010).

# Recent Developments in Primary Care Reforms in Canada

## COLLABORATIVE CARE

Collaborative care based on interaction and shared knowledge, expertise, and decision-making processes among different health care providers has been shown to reduce service duplication and health care costs, improve access to primary care services, improve health outcomes, and increase patient and provider satisfaction (Health Canada, 2007a). Additionally, collaborative primary care teams are thought to be better positioned to focus on health promotion, chronic disease prevention and management (Chan & Wood, 2010; Health Canada, 2007a), and to provide holistic, higher quality care than physicians working in solo practices (Statistics Canada, 2008). The benefits of team approaches have been identified by both female providers and users of the health care system in the US (Peters, 2010) and are in line with the reported value that women place on care that incorporates psychological health, family, and relationships (Hills & Mullett, 2005). Collaborative care is also preferred by female physicians who, along with younger physicians, represent the main adopters of team approaches in Canada (College of Family Physicians of Canada, Canadian Medical Association & Royal College of Physicians and Surgeons of Canada, 2007). A unique study comparing primary care service models in Ontario and their differential impact on women and men showed that community health centres, which are largely based on collaborative care, had the "smallest gender gap and best performance for women" (Dahrouge et al., 2010, 8), in terms of receiving prevention services and being recommended care for chronic diseases (Dahrouge et al., 2010).

To date, most primary health care teams in Canada are largely physician-led (College of Family Physicians of Canada et al., 2007), but it has been noted that the composition of teams is important. Teams with greater occupational diversity have higher overall effectiveness and greater impact on patient care (Borrill, West, Shapiro & Rees, 2000). Changes in the mix of providers offering primary care, both in terms of a wider range of providers and the gender balance among providers, have led to new opportunities for women as providers and users of primary care. Women have made significant inroads into the previously male-dominated field of medicine and dominate professions such as nursing, midwifery, and nurse practitioners (NPs). Women are also beginning to challenge the male domination among physician assistants (PAs) in Canada, where current female enrolment rates at Canadian universities are as high as 86 percent (Danielle Laffan, personal communication, October 14, 2010). Referring to a literature review by Wilson and Childs from 2003, Kringos and colleagues argue that "the gender balance of the primary care workforce can influence access, continuity and efficiency of care, and the scope of services available" (2010, 6). Thus we can expect to see changes in primary care as more women enter new areas of professional practice.

## PATIENT-CENTRED CARE

The concept of patient-centred care has received significant attention since the release of the US Institute of Medicine's *Crossing the Quality Chasm* in 2001, which identified patient-centred care as one of the six aims of high-quality care. The Institute of Medicine defined patient-centred care as care that is "respectful of and responsive to individual patient preferences, needs and values, and ensuring that patient values guide all clinical decisions" (Institute of Medicine 2001 in Epstein, Fiscella, Lesser & Stange, 2010, 1489). It is built on relationships among physicians, patients, and patients' families through dialogue, engagement, information sharing, and trust. Patient-centred care has been shown to improve disease-related outcomes and quality of life, as well as to reduce costs and address racial, ethnic, and socioeconomic disparities in care and outcomes in the US (Epstein et al., 2010).

While there may be variations in the model of patient-centred care, models that encourage patients to participate, question, and be decision-makers in their own health care may align well with women's interests and could also have a positive impact on underserved populations by addressing their barriers in accessing care, such as illiteracy, language, and cultural barriers (Silow-Carroll, Alteras & Stepnick, 2006). According to Hills and Mullett (2005), for example, women are more interested than men in making informed decisions and being partners in health care decision-making. On the provider side, research suggests that female providers are more likely than male providers to spend time interacting with their patients (Ahmad, Stewart, Cameron & Hyman, 2001; Roter & Hall, 2004) and also have a less dominant interaction style with their patients (Schmid Mast, 2004). Roter and Hall (2004) found that female physicians are more likely to exhibit patient-centred behaviours because their medical visits were longer and they "engaged in more active partnership behaviours, positive talk, psychosocial counseling, psychosocial question asking, and emotionally focused talk" (Roter & Hall, 2004, 497). Further, the authors found that "patient behavior largely reciprocates gender-linked physician behaviors" (p. 510) so that patients of female physicians tend to talk more, share more psychosocial information, and build partnerships.

Such differences in interaction may have an impact on health outcomes and quality of care. For example, Bean-Mayberry and colleagues (2006) and Franks and Bertakis (2003) suggest that patients with female providers are more likely to receive gender-specific preventive care and routine gynecologic and mammography services than patients with male providers. However, investigations into gendered patterns of some procedures, such as total joint arthroplasty, suggest that there is a need to investigate further whether there are gender biases in referral patterns for some procedures (Jackson, Pederson & Boscoe, 2009). There is some support, therefore, for the notion that patient-centred care, with its focus on identifying patient needs and preferences, and its emphasis on the patient-provider relationship, may be an

important development advance for women's care recipients—
though it needs to be sharpened with equity analyses that examine issues of gender, diversity, and intersectionality if it is to be
truly relevant to women's (and indeed, men's) needs.

## CHRONIC CONDITION PREVENTION AND MANAGEMENT

Calls for addressing the prevention and management of chronic
conditions have become increasingly loud in Canada (Health Canada, 2007b, n.d.-b; Swerissen, 2008; VanSoeren et al., 2008). Caring for chronic conditions requires mechanisms for monitoring
patients who need regular tests, strategies for fostering collaborative decision-making processes for medication use and treatment
plans, and an overall adjustment in the patient-provider relationship from episodic to regular contact. The Chronic Care Model
(Wagner et al., 2002) and the British Columbia Expanded Chronic
Care Model (Barr et al., 2003), for example, identify essential elements in chronic disease management as "prepared, proactive
practice teams," "informed, activated patients" (Barr et al., 2003;
Wagner et al., 2002), "prepared, proactive community partners,"
an "activated community," healthy public policy, and supportive
environments (Barr et al., 2003).

In view of the rates of chronic conditions among women, a focus
on chronic condition prevention and management is both welcome
and necessary to improve women's health. However, traditional
approaches to chronic disease management have not always been
sensitive to the particular realities of women's lives (Anderson, Dyck
& Lynam, 1997). Self-management programs have had some positive effects over the short term, such as increased self-efficacy and
self-rated health (Jovicic, Leduc & Straus, 2006; Norris, Engelgau
& Narayan, 2001; Warsi, Wang, LaValley, Avorn & Solomon, 2004),
but there is a concern that current self-management policy and
practice directions could "increase rather than ameliorate health
inequities" (Mills, Osborne, Brady, Rogers & Vanden, 2009). Marginalized groups are not gaining access to programs, and program
content has often been shown to be irrelevant and inappropriate to

the lives of some of those suffering from chronic conditions. This is particularly true of disadvantaged individuals because self-management programs often do not account for the diverse experiences of women and men managing illness and tend to overlook the role of social determinants of health (Mills et al., 2009).

Despite the number of innovations that have been introduced in the last 40 years in Canada, Hutchison and colleagues (2001) contend that we have scarcely seen even incremental change in the system of primary care. Further, a recent poll conducted on behalf of the Canadian Medical Association showed that nine in 10 Canadians believe that they have not seen any real solutions being put forward by governments (Ipsos Reid, 2010). Government, health care providers, researchers, patients, and the general public have long expressed their concern with the Canadian health system's accessibility, responsiveness, continuity of care, and lack of holistic approach (Wong, Watson, Young & Regan, 2008). The recent developments presented in this chapter, which represent only a few examples, provide some hope for women as providers and users of primary care. However, a more deliberate, women-centred approach to primary care reform might combine all three features of primary care reform — collaborative care, patient-centred care, and chronic condition prevention and management — with a gender lens to produce a model of primary care reform that works better for women.

# Developing a Women-Centred Approach to Primary Care

Both sex-specific and gendered factors shape women's needs for primary care. Women require birth control, prenatal, childbirth, and postnatal care, routine care for menstruation and menopause, female infertility, and periodic cervical cancer screening. Women also need care for diseases for which they have a higher prevalence than men, such as breast cancer, eating disorders, depression, and self-inflicted injuries, as well as conditions that appear to be sex-neutral, but whose signs, symptoms, and treatment methods might differ between women and men. In addition to these sex-specific needs within primary care, women's caring responsibilities often require them to seek out care for dependent children, people with disabilities, and others with acute or chronic illness (Pederson & Donner, 2007). Thus, women's needs for, and experiences of, primary care are both distinct from and overlap with those of men's, and are influenced by the context of care and assumptions, beliefs, and experiences of health care providers, not simply medical need.

When it comes to reproductive health screening, an Australian study suggests that women "are seeking a woman friendly and women-centred service, a safe environment and continuity of care" (Peters, 2010, 2557). Many women also want to be able to choose their provider and/or setting for primary care (Peters, 2010); in some cases, this means finding a provider who shares their cultural experience or language (Marshall, Wong, Haggerty & Levesque, 2010; O'Malley, Forrest & O'Malley, 2000) and it often means having a female provider perform reproductive screening procedures (i.e., breast and cervical cancer screening). A systematic literature review by Jung and colleagues (2003) showed that younger patients had a "more marked preference for a female physician" than older patients (p. 168), and young women preferred a different physician from their parents. Female patients also preferred consultations with nurses over doctors and valued thorough examinations, screening for cancer, and preventive care (Jung et al., 2003). A Canadian study showed that older women are more concerned about living with disabilities than with common diseases, and value care that focuses on health maintenance strategies, active participation in health promotion, and injury prevention (Tannenbaum & Mayo, 2003). A study on First Nations women's experiences with health care showed that their health concerns are often dismissed by providers. First Nations women were often met with racialized and gendered stereotypes that influenced the health care they received and made them reluctant to seek care until symptoms were severe, resulting in poor health outcomes (Browne & Fiske, 2001). This is particularly worrisome in view of First Nations women's higher incidence of diabetes, tobacco addiction, and HIV/AIDS compared to other women in Canada (Mann, 2005), and highlights the importance of accessible, equitable, and culturally appropriate health care for all women.

With respect to access to services, women often experience more and different barriers in accessing health care than men, including limited financial resources, and caregiving and child-rearing responsibilities (Hills & Mullett, 2005), which need to be considered in designing care. Women have also called for a primary care system where they can receive quality care that goes beyond reproductive health, incorporating psychological health, social functioning, sexual health, and relationships (Hills & Mullett, 2005). Studies in the US have shown that low-income women want primary care to be convenient with respect to location, accessible by public transport, and open during convenient hours, especially on evenings and weekends (O'Malley & Forrest, 2002; O'Malley et al., 2000). In addition, it has been shown that women value continuity of care (particularly with a single clinician), the physician-patient relationship, a comprehensive scope of service, coordination between providers, and accountability (O'Malley et al., 2000). These results are consistent with research in Canada that demonstrates that low-income Canadians experience barriers to care that influence their use of health services (e.g., Williamson et al., 2006). Thus care that paid attention to women and women's needs would be organized in ways that do not perpetuate the disadvantages some women experience in accessing care by, for example, providing supports for transportation to care, being open evenings and weekends (O'Malley & Forrest, 2002; O'Malley et al., 2000) and making provisions for women to bring their children to appointments if necessary (Hills & Mullett, 2005).

Initiatives that fail to consider a patient's social context in the management and prevention of chronic conditions may have negative effects on women. Eakin and colleagues (2002) highlight that people living in underserved communities, people with low income, and ethnic minority populations often face barriers in implementing and accessing management and prevention programs. Gender-based differences in access to, comfort with, and use of chronic condition prevention and management programs therefore must be considered in the design, implementation, and evaluation of these programs to create a range of effective programs able to meet the diverse goals and needs of women (Mills et al., 2009).

Similar conclusions were reached by participants of a workshop sponsored by Women and Health Care Reform in early 2004 (Pederson & Jackson, 2004). The central conclusion of the workshop was that much of the discussion of primary care reform in official circles was focused on managerial issues such as the specifics of funding and the organization and delivery of care, but that if reforms were really to benefit women, they should embrace the primary *health* care approach articulated in the Alma Ata Declaration (Pederson & Jackson, 2004). This position was subsequently shared at the first-ever National Primary Health Care Summit in May 2004. A discussion paper by Donner and Pederson (2004), prepared for the workshop and subsequently published in the *Journal of the Pan American Health Organization* (Pederson & Donner, 2007), argued that in keeping with the spirit of primary *health* care, decision-makers and health care providers need to recognize the importance of women's diverse social locations and the context of their lives in order to understand and address women's access to, and needs for, primary care. They suggested that no single model of primary care services would serve all women, but that a women-centred approach to the design and implementation of primary care reforms would help care not only to be accessible but also acceptable to women. Workshop participants also urged decision-makers to see primary care reform as a process, not an outcome, and to recognize the value and centrality of relationships in the dynamics between women and health care providers (Pederson & Jackson, 2004).

Gregor (1997) argues that the shift in the past 20 years to greater care in the community, a greater reliance on ambulatory care, and increased responsibility for chronic disease management at the level of primary care "must necessarily affect women to a greater degree than men" (p. 30) because these three trends rely on women to provide informal, unpaid care at home. Despite these numerous changes, it is rare that primary care and primary care reforms reflect women's health care needs or are organized with women in mind.

In fact, Weisman and colleagues (2010) have suggested that care that is designed based on girls' and women's needs and preferences regarding care, and that recognizes the importance of social location in shaping women's access to care, as well as capacities for managing their own health, holds promise as a model for providing primary care not only for women but for everyone else. Women-centred care explicitly acknowledges the influence of gender on the need for and experience of care (Hills & Mullett, 2002), paying attention both to the biological factors of the female body and the social conditions of girls' and women's lives that shape their access to, preferences for, and experiences of care.

Hills and Mullett (2002) have identified eight guiding principles for women-centred care (see box). There is some research available to support women-centred primary care, though little from Canada and no ongoing support for continued examination of this approach. For example, evaluations of the US Centers of Excellence (Anderson et al., 2001; Weisman, Curbow & Khoury, 1995; Weisman & Squires, 2000), funded by the US Department of Health and Human Services to "develop standards for comprehensive, multidisciplinary, and culturally competent approaches to women's health across the life-span" (Anderson et al., 2002, 310), demonstrate that these centres provide more screening tests and counselling services than in other primary care settings, and that patients report higher levels of care satisfaction than women served elsewhere. Various models have been used in these centres, including a "one-stop shopping" model in which a comprehensive array of services is co-located in a single facility, and a "centres without walls" model in which services are networked together, but provided in different sites. While the results of comprehensive evaluation studies of these sites were promising, "there is little evidence that the models of care embodied by the National Centers of Excellence diffused to other primary care settings serving the general U.S. population or has been further evaluated" (Weisman et al., 2010, 229). Federal funding for the centres has now been discontinued (Weisman et al., 2010), which is discouraging news given the positive findings from the evaluation studies, and it represents a backward step in women's health for the US. In Canada, evaluations of existing initiatives are also needed, as are reviews of promising research for information on women and gender in relation to primary care and primary care reform. The study by Dahrouge and colleagues (2010), comparing different models of primary care practices in Ontario in relation to gender mentioned previously, suggests that different organizational models (fee for service, community health centres, family health networks, and health service organizations) provide somewhat different services to women and men. Specifically, the authors documented gender-related inequities in chronic disease care and in health promotion discussions between providers and patients, depending on the model of care. More studies of this sort are needed to further develop our understanding of the relationship between care model and appropriate provision of men's and women's health needs in Canada.

## BOX 2.1: Guiding Principles for Women-Centred Care (Hills & Mullett, 2002, 92)

1. Treat women with respect. This includes preserving women's dignity, accepting women's knowledge of their being, and acknowledging their experiences.
2. Acknowledge and accept the diversity of women. Diversity includes physiology, ethnicity, economic circumstances, sexual orientation, ability, culture, religion, and level of education.
3. Acknowledge women as the predominant caregivers who very often provide the safety net for others in our society. In addition, recognize that women experience greater difficulty with access to health care because of their childrearing and caregiving responsibilities.
4. Actively explore and consider the impacts of the social, economic, societal, and environmental factors on women's lives. Recognize the gender imbalances in our society and other cultures.
5. Give women information to facilitate their making informed choices. Women will be encouraged to exercise their right to ask questions and will be provided with the opportunity to consider appropriate alternative therapies.
6. When appropriate, seek cooperation with mutually supportive health professionals in order to promote synergistic collaboration, continuity, and quality of care.
7. Allow self determination to manage the issue of whether or not family members or significant others will be in attendance during consultations.
8. Consider the possible contributions that other health care providers may make, including those whose approaches are other than mainstream medicine.

In addition to these guiding principles, we suggest that women-centred care should be informed by research into women's preferences for care, as well as by evidence of women's experiences of illness, and evaluations of demonstration projects and/or innovative approaches to delivering primary care. Despite its name, women-centred care needs to pay attention to more than issues of sex and gender as a comprehensive understanding of women's health recognizes the importance of other determinants of health, including income, race, education, age, and language (Hankivsky, 2006). As Brittle and Bird observe,

> The gender-based medicine objective fits within a larger effort aimed at creating evidence-based medical care and one aimed at delivering patient-centered care. However, gender differences in healthcare needs extend beyond a simple disparities model. Unlike racial/ethnic and socio-economic disparities in care, gender differences in health-care needs, and in quality of care, are related to both social and biological factors that affect men's and women's health, healthcare utilization, and outcomes of care. (2007, 143)

Moreover, a fully realized model of women-centred primary care will necessarily involve attending to the interface between the health care system and other determinants of health, and will serve as the starting point for a discussion of women's health care needs across the life course and stages of care, from primary care to long-term and residential care.

# Conclusion

In the US, Weisman and colleagues (2010) have suggested that a primary care system that is designed with women in mind will likely benefit all users of primary care because a fully women-centred primary care system would solve the issues of access, fragmentation, and silos of care that plague primary care in the US. While the Canadian primary care system may have fewer access problems than the US because of our model of universal public health insurance, we nevertheless have documented barriers to care, issues of fragmentation, and a lack of coordination of care (Starfield, 2010).

Research into women-specific aspects of primary care and some of the directions of primary care reform in Canada give us reasons to be somewhat hopeful about the evolution of primary care in this country. The articulation and evaluation of women-centred care approaches, in particular, come close to fulfilling many of the elements of *primary health care* that were articulated by the WHO; indeed, Hills and Mullett (2005) argue that primary health care is the preferred service delivery option for women. While we would agree, we also share the concern of Vlassoff and Moreno (2002) that even the WHO version of primary health care "was promoted without adequate consideration of gender" (p. 1714). In fact, we share their concern that some versions of primary health care have tended to perpetuate some aspects of gender roles. To illustrate, Vlassoff and Moreno describe many primary health care programs that have "perpetuated the notion that child care is almost exclusively a woman's role" (2002, 1714), and argue that some of the activities associated with primary health care require large time commitments from women without offering visible benefits or results (Vlassoff & Moreno, 2002). Thus some versions of primary health care have maintained or relied upon traditional gendered patterns of household labour and inadvertently devalued women's time and effort, with the unintended effect of weakening some women's commitment to primary care reforms (Vlassoff & Moreno, 2002).

Without a critical gender analysis, calls for primary health care as the preferred outcome of primary care reform continue to run the risk of perpetuating rather than reforming the dominant ideological and structural underpinnings of primary care in Canada, thus constraining rather than enhancing women as users, providers, and decision-makers in primary care. We suggest that research examining the innovations that have been undertaken with respect to women's primary care, including facilities that explicitly aim to implement women-centred care, is needed. In its ideal form, women-centred care corresponds closely to the principles and aspirations of primary health care, but reinterprets that vision through the lens of gender and gender equity. The vision of primary health care — and, in particular, its call for alignment between primary care and the determinants of health — is not enough (Rasanathan et al., 2010). Truly innovative primary care in Canada will integrate the best of the primary health care model with the principles and knowledge gained from a critical commitment to women-centred care.

## Note

1. The term "chronic condition" is increasingly being used instead of "chronic disease," acknowledging the distinction between disease processes and other forms of impairment, such as chronic pain and some forms of disability (Mills et al., 2009).

## References

Ahmad, F., Stewart, D.E., Cameron, J.I. & Hyman, I. (2001). Rural physicians' perspectives on cervical and breast cancer screening: A gender-based analysis. *Journal of Women's Health & Gender-Based Medicine 10*(2), 201–208.

Anderson, J., Dyck, I. & Lynam, J. (1997). Health care professionals and women speaking: Constraints in everyday life and the management of chronic illness. *Health 1*, 57–80.

Anderson, R., Barbara, A., Weisman, C., Scholle, S., Binko, J., Schneider, T., et al. (2001). A qualitative analysis of women's satisfaction with primary care from a panel of focus groups in the national centers of excellence in women's health. *Journal of Women's Health & Gender-Based Medicine 10*(7), 637–647.

Anderson, R., Weisman, C., Hudson Scholle, S., Henderson, J., Olden-dick, R. & Camacho, F. (2002). *Evaluation of the quality of care in the clinical care centers of the national centers of excellence in women's health.* Retrieved from http://64.94.16.210/owh/multidisciplinary/coe/journals/AndersonArticle1.pdf

Armstrong, P. & Armstrong, H. (2008). *Health care.* Black Point: Fernwood.

Barer, M. (2002). New opportunities for old mistakes. *Health Affairs* 21(1), 169–171.

Barr, V.J., Robinson, S., Marin-Link, B., Underhill, L., Dotts, A., Ravens-dale, D., et al. (2003). The expanded chronic care model: An integration of concepts and strategies from population health promotion and the chronic care model. *Hospital Quarterly* 7(1), 73–82.

Bean-Mayberry, B.A., Chang, C.-C.H., McNeil, M.A. & HudsonScholle, S. (2006). Ensuring high-quality primary care for women: Predictors of success. *Women's Health Issues* 16(1), 22–29.

Beaulieu, M.-D., Rioux, M., Rocher, G., Samson, L. & Boucher, L. (2008). Family practice: Professional identity in transition. A case study of family medicine in Canada. *Social Science & Medicine 67*, 1153–1163.

Borrill, C., West, M., Shapiro, D. & Rees, A. (2000). Team working and effectiveness in health care. *British Journal of Health Care Management 6*(8), 364–371.

Brittle, C. & Bird, C.E. (2007). *Literature review on effective sex- and gender-based systems/models of care.* Retrieved from http://www.womenshealth.gov/owh/multidisciplinary/reports/GenderBasedMedicine/FinalOWHReport.pdf

Browne, A.J. & Fiske, J.-A. (2001). First Nations women's encounters with mainstream health care services. *Western Journal of Nursing Research* 23(2), 126–147.

Chan, A.K. & Wood, V. (2010). Preparing tomorrow's healthcare providers for interprofessional collaborative patient-centred practice today. *UBC Medical Journal* 1(2), 22–24.

College of Family Physicians of Canada, Canadian Medical Association & Royal College of Physicians and Surgeons of Canada. (2007). *2007 National physician survey.*

Dahrouge, S., Hogg, W., Tuna, M., Russell, G., Devlin, R., Tugwell, P., et al. (2010). An evaluation of gender equity in different models of primary care practices in Ontario. *BMC Public Health 10*(151).

Donner, L. & Pederson, A. (2004). *Beyond vectors and vessels: Women and primary health care reform in Canada.* Toronto: Women and Health Care Reform.

Eakin, E.G., Bull, S.S., Glasgow, R.E. & Mason, M. (2002). Reaching those most in need: A review of diabetes self-management interventions in disadvantaged populations. *Diabetes/Metabolism Research and Reviews 18*, 26–35.

Epstein, R.M., Fiscella, K., Lesser, C.S. & Stange, K.C. (2010). Why the nation needs a policy push on patient-centered health care. *Health Affairs 29*(8), 1489–1495.

Evans, R. & McGrail, K. (2008). Richard III, Barer-Stoddart, and the daughter of time. *Healthcare Policy 3*(3), 18–28.

Franks, P. & Bertakis, K.D. (2003). Physician gender, patient gender, and primary care. *Journal of Women's Health 12*(1), 73.

Gregor, F. (1997). From women to women: Nurses, informal caregivers, and the gender dimension of health care reform in Canada. *Health and Social Care in the Community 5*(1), 30–36.

Hankivsky, O. (2006). Beijing and beyond: Women's health and gender-based analysis in Canada. *International Journal of Health Services 36*(2), 377–400.

Health Canada. (2007a). *Primary health care transition fund: Collaborative care.* Retrieved from http://www.hc-sc.gc.ca/hcs-sss/alt_formats/hpb-dgps/pdf/prim/2006-synth-collabor-eng.pdf

Health Canada. (2007b). *Primary health care transition fund: Chronic disease prevention and management.* Ottawa: Health Canada.

Health Canada. (2007c). *Primary health care transition fund: Summary of initiatives.* Ottawa: Health Canada.

Health Canada. (n.d.-a). *2003 First ministers' accord on health care renewal.* Retrieved from http://www.hc-sc.gc.ca/hcs-sss/delivery-prestation/fptcollab/2003accord/index-eng.php

Health Canada. (n.d.-b). *About primary health care.* Retrieved from http://www.hc-sc.gc.ca/hcs-sss/prim/about-apropos-eng.php

Health Council of Canada. (2010). At the tipping point: Health leaders share ideas to speed primary health care reform. Retrieved from http://www.healthcouncilcanada.ca/docs/rpts/2010/HCC_Commentary_pages2_052510.pdf

Hills, M. & Mullett, J. (2002). Women-centred care: Working collaboratively to develop gender inclusive health policy. *Health Care for Women International* 23(1), 84–97.

Hills, M. & Mullett, J. (2005). Primary health care: A preferred health service delivery option for women. *Health Care for Women International* 26, 325–339.

Hutchison, B. (2008). A long time coming: Primary healthcare renewal in Canada. [Invited essay.] *HealthcarePapers* 8(2), 10–24.

Hutchison, B., Abelson, J. & Lavis, J. (2001). Primary care in Canada: So much innovation, so little change. *Health Affairs* 20(3), 116–131.

Ipsos Reid. (2010). *Canadians to Prime Minister Harper: Don't forget about healthcare.* Ottawa: Ipsos Reid.

Jackson, B.E., Pederson, A. & Boscoe, M. (2009). Waiting to wait: Improving wait times evidence through gender-based analysis. In P. Armstrong & J. Deadman (Eds.), *Women's health: Intersections of policy, research, and practice* (pp. 35–51). Toronto: Women's Press.

Jovicic, A., Leduc, J.H. & Straus, S. (2006). Effects of self-management intervention on health outcomes of patients with heart failure: A systematic review of randomized controlled trials. *BMC Cardiovascular Disorders* 6(43).

Jung, H.P., Baerveldt, C., Olesen, F., Grol, R. & Wensing, M. (2003). Patient characteristics as predictors of primary health care preferences: A systematic literature analysis. *Health Expectations* 6(2), 160–181.

Keleher, H. (2001). Why primary health care offers a more comprehensive approach to tackling health inequities than primary care. *Australian Journal of Primary Health* 7(2), 57–61.

Kringos, D., Boerma, W., Hutchinson, A., van der Zee, J. & Groenewegen, P. (2010). The breadth of primary care: A systematic literature review of its core dimensions. *BMC Health Services Research* 10(1), 65.

Mann, M. (2005). *Aboriginal women: An issues backgrounder.* Retrieved from http://www.michellemann.ca/articles/Aboriginal%20Women%20-%20An%20Issues%20Backgrounder.pdf

Marshall, E., Wong, S., Haggerty, J. & Levesque, J. (2010). Perceptions of unmet healthcare needs: What do Punjabi and Chinese-speaking immigrants think? A qualitative study. *BMC Health Services Research 10*, 46–53.

Mills, S., Osborne, R., Brady, T., Rogers, A. & Vanden, E. (2009). *The international roundtable on self-management of chronic conditions: Summary report, "Minding the gap": Building a framework to bridge evidence, policy, and practice in chronic disease self-management.* Vancouver: BC Centre of Excellence for Women's Health.

Norris, S., Engelgau, M. & Narayan, K. (2001). Effectiveness of self-management training in type 2 diabetes: A systematic review of randomized controlled trials. *Diabetes Care 24*(3), 561–587.

O'Malley, A. & Forrest, C. (2002). The mismatch between urban women's preferences for and experiences with primary care. *Women's Health Issues 12*(4), 191–203.

O'Malley, A., Forrest, C. & O'Malley, P. (2000). Low-income women's priorities for primary care. *Journal of Family Practice 49*(2), 141–146.

Pederson, A. & Donner, L. (2007). Beyond vectors and vessels: Reflections on women and primary health care reform in Canada. *Pan American Journal of Public Health 21*(2/3), 145–154.

Pederson, A. & Jackson, B.E. (2004). *Dare to dream: Reflections on a national workshop on women and primary health care.* Toronto: Women and Health Care Reform.

Peters, K. (2010). Reasons why women choose a medical practice or a women's health centre for routine health screening: Worker and client perspectives. *Journal of Clinical Nursing 19*(17–18), 2557–2564.

Rasanathan, K., Montesinos, E., Matheson, D., Etienne, C. & Evans, T. (2010). Primary health care and the social determinants of health: Essential and complementary approaches for reducing inequities in health. *Journal of Epidemiology and Community Health.* 65(8), 656–60.

Romanow, R.J. (2002). *Building on values: The future of health care in Canada.* Saskatoon. Commission on the Future of Health Care in Canada.

Roter, D.L. & Hall, J.A. (2004). Physician gender and patient-centered communication: A critical review of empirical research. *Annual Review of Public Health 25*(1), 497–519.

Schmid Mast, M. (2004). Dominance and gender in the physician-patient interaction. *Journal of Men's Health & Gender* 1(4), 354–358.

Silow-Carroll, S., Alteras, T. & Stepnick, L. (2006). *Patient-centered care for underserved populations: Definition and best practices*. Washington: Economical Social Research Institute.

Starfield, B. (2010). Reinventing primary care: Lessons from Canada for the United States. *Health Affairs* 29(5), 1030–1036.

Statistics Canada. (2008). *Primary health care teams and their impact on processes and outcomes of care*. Ottawa: Statistics Canada.

Swerissen, H. (2008). Rethinking primary healthcare. *HealthcarePapers* 8(2), 54–57.

Tannenbaum, C. & Mayo, N. (2003). Women's health priorities and perceptions of care: A survey to identify opportunities for improving preventative health care delivery for older women. *Age and Ageing* 32(6), 626–635.

Thurston, W. & O'Connor, M. (1996). *Health promotion for women*. Paper prepared for the Canada–USA Forum on Women's Health. Ottawa: Health Canada.

VanSoeren, M., Hurlock-Chorostecki, C., Pogue, P. & Sanders, J. (2008). Primary healthcare renewal in Canada: A glass half empty? *HealthcarePapers* 8(2), 39–44.

Vlassoff, C. & Moreno, C.G. (2002). Placing gender at the centre of health programming: Challenges and limitations. *Social Science & Medicine* 54, 1713–1723.

Wagner, E., Davis, C., Schaefer, J., Von Korff, M. & Austin, B. (2002). A survey of leading chronic disease management programs: Are they consistent with the literature? *Journal of Nursing Care Quality* 16(2), 67–80.

Warsi, A., Wang, P., LaValley, M., Avorn, J. & Solomon, D. (2004). Self-management education programs in chronic disease: A systematic review and methodological critique of the literature. *Archives of Internal Medicine* 164, 1641–1649.

Watson, D. & McGrail, K. (2009). More doctors or better care? *Healthcare Policy* 5(1), 26–31.

Weatherill, S. (2007). *Laying the groundwork for culture change: The legacy of the primary health care transition fund*. Retrieved from http://www.

hc-sc.gc.ca/hcs-sss/alt_formats/hpb-dgps/pdf/prim/2006-synth-legacy-fondements-eng.pdf

Webster, P.C. (2010). CIHR pledges to tackle primary health care. *Canadian Medical Association Journal 182*(4), E188–189.

Weisman, C.S., Chuang, C.H. & Scholle, S.H. (2010). Still piecing it together: Women's primary care. *Women's Health Issues 20*(4), 228–230.

Weisman, C.S., Curbow, B. & Khoury, A.J. (1995). The national survey of women's health centers: Current models of women-centered care. *Women's Health Issues 5*(3), 103–117.

Weisman, C.S. & Squires, G.L. (2000). Women's health centers: Are the national centers of excellence in women's health a new model? *Women's Health Issues 10*(5), 248–255.

Williamson, D., Stewart, M., Hayward, K., Letourneau, N., Makwarimba, E., Masudab, J., et al. (2006). Low-income Canadians' experiences with health-related services: Implications for health care reform. *Health Policy 76*, 106–121.

Women and Health Care Reform. (n.d). Women and health care reform group. Retrieved from http://www.womenandhealthcarereform.ca/

Wong, S., Watson, D., Young, E. & Regan, S. (2008). What do people think is important about primary healthcare? *Healthcare Policy 3*(3), 89–104.

World Health Organization. (2008). *The world health report 2008: Primary health care now more than ever.* Geneva: WHO.

World Health Organization. (n.d.). *Declaration of Alma-Ata.* Retrieved from http://www.who.int/hpr/NPH/docs/declaration_almaata.pdf

CHAPTER 3

# Assembling the Evidence for Thinking Women

BETH JACKSON, ANN PEDERSON, AND MORGAN SEELEY

## Introduction

Health researchers and policy actors need to summarize and synthesize evidence to clarify what is known about health systems and policies, to identify what evidence gaps exists, and to inform future research and action (Popay & Roberts, 2006). Over the last 20 years, demands for more scientifically rigorous ways of synthesizing evidence have given rise to evidence-based decision-making and practice, particularly in the fields of medicine and health care, and have prompted the development of numerous evidence review and synthesis methods. In health research, many types of evidence synthesis are practised, but the dominant approach—epitomized by the methods of the Cochrane Collaboration and often described as the "gold standard" for evidence reviews—is most concerned with the effectiveness of interventions, i.e., Did the intervention cause the intended outcome? However, health policy and intervention research goes beyond effectiveness to ask other key questions, like *why* and *how* does a policy/intervention work (or not), *for whom*, and *in what circumstances?* Because of the complex interdependencies of social structures and relationships, because of the multiple contextual factors that can affect an intervention or policy, and because of long time lags between intervention and effect, causal relationships are often difficult to demonstrate for interventions in "real-world" circumstances. Accordingly, researchers and policy actors need to draw upon a wide range of data, evidence, and methods of synthesis.

In this chapter, we explore the capacity of dominant and emerging systematic review methods to address women's experiences of health interventions. We ask: What evidence-based review strategies are available for research and decision-making in health? What strategies are needed to assess evidence for complex health interventions? What are the limitations of dominant methods of systematic review? And, given our commitment to documenting the impact of health care reforms on women's lives across a range of social locations, how might realist reviews (as one emerging approach to evidence synthesis) address these limitations and advance the goals of sex- and gender-based analysis (SGBA) and equity-based research and decision-making? We ask these questions in reference to a pressing and persistent health policy concern: wait times for medical and surgical interventions. Specifically, our evidence reviews focus on the impact of sex and gender on hip- and knee-replacement surgery wait times.

## Systematic Evidence Reviews in Health Research, Policy, and Practice

Evidence reviews enable us to summarize large amounts of evidence on a topic, which is crucial in health policy and health services research where accumulation of new evidence is increasingly rapid. According to Pope, Mays, and Popay (2007), the synthesis of findings from multiple studies can improve understanding of phenomena, identify gaps in the research, and stimulate new research questions. This "should not be taken to mean that research syntheses are necessarily a more accurate reflection of the true state of affairs than any one study, but simply that they afford opportunities for comparison and cumulation which are not possible with a single study, however robust" (Mays, Roberts & Popay, 2001, 190). Nevertheless, where policy and treatment decisions must be made on the best available evidence, systematic reviews are important tools for policy actors and health care providers.

The term "systematic review" is used to describe a wide range of methods for reviewing and synthesizing evidence. It emerged in the context of clinical treatment and its application has a relatively short history in the sphere of public health and health care policy, yet an expanding array of approaches, methods, and foci for evidence review and synthesis have emerged in recent years. Systematic reviews and syntheses examine the effectiveness of (clinical) interventions, and support decision-making about interventions; for example, by examining cost effectiveness, the diversity and distribution of policy impact, and the delivery and implementation of interventions (Mays, Pope & Popay, 2005; Popay & Roberts, 2006). Common approaches to evidence review and synthesis include, but are not limited to, Cochrane Collaboration and Campbell Collaboration reviews, scoping reviews, rapid evidence assessments, systematic narrative reviews, meta-ethnography, case survey methods, Bayesian meta-analysis, and realist reviews (Centre for Reviews & Dissemination, 2009; Dixon-Woods, Agarwal, Jones, Young & Sutton, 2005; Mays, Pope & Popay, 2005; Sandelowski, Docherty & Emden, 1997). The scope of this chapter permits only a brief review of key methods for reviews and syntheses.

Different systematic review approaches reflect different purposes, such as reviews aimed at providing knowledge support or those used to support decision-making (Mays, Pope & Popay, 2005). Assorted methods address different research/policy/management questions (e.g., presence/size of a problem, intervention effectiveness, intervention costs), and may require different types of evidence (e.g., evidence from randomized controlled trials [RCTs] vs. observational evidence). Nevertheless, as mentioned above, most reviews focus on questions of intervention effectiveness, and it has been argued that "methods for reviewing and synthesising other types of evidence to address questions beyond effectiveness remain much less well developed" (Popay & Roberts, 2006, 1).

Despite a wide range of approaches to systematically reviewing and synthesizing evidence in the health field, the dominant or conventional systematic review methodology and paradigm remains the Cochrane Collaboration approach. This approach focuses on assessing intervention effectiveness (Bambra, 2009; Shepperd et al., 2009) by pooling, synthesizing, and presenting evidence to address a pre-specified research question using an explicit and reproducible methodology (see Higgins & Green, 2008). Conventional Cochrane-style systematic reviews are often (sometimes inappropriately) used as a standard against which narrative reviews are judged. Narrative reviews summarize studies through a systematic process of defining key terms, scoping the literature, and selecting relevant studies. They may draw on the subjective knowledge, experience, and expertise of authors/ reviewers and tend to be receptive to a variety of evidence types (e.g., qualitative and quantitative, qualitative only, key informant interviews, etc.). Narrative reviews generally try to answer the "how" and "why" questions (explanatory) rather than to ask *if* an intervention works or not (effectiveness questions).

Conventional systematic review techniques have traditionally excluded non-experimental, qualitative, and other forms of evidence, and have been applied in error to reviews that have required a critical analysis of a complex body of literature (see Dixon-Woods et al., 2005, 2006). This is especially relevant to analysis of data and evidence that may shed light on equity concerns, and has led some scholars to express concern about the potentially harmful consequences of reviews that lack sex- and gender-based and other equity-focused analyses. Commenting on the dominant paradigm's "track record" on equity analysis, Boscoe, Tudiver, Doull, and Runnels note that "despite guidelines that encourage researchers to include demographic and other population characteristics, various studies of systematic reviews have revealed a lack of adequate attention to health equity factors, including sex and gender" (2009, 44). In the current culture of evidence-based decision-making in health systems and policy arenas, and in the context of federal policies that both support and require SGBA analysis of programs and policies, this is a significant gap. To help address this gap, the Cochrane Health Equity Field is presently collaborating with a group of experts in SGBA to develop and test a *Sex and Gender Appraisal Tool* for systematic reviews (see Boscoe, Tudiver, Doull & Runnels, 2009), but significant challenges to its uptake remain.

**WHAT EVIDENCE REVIEWS ARE NEEDED?**
Health, health systems, and policy/program interventions are complex; their study crosses many research disciplines and methodological approaches and creates a wide range of data and evidence. Experts in health-focused knowledge translation and exchange have asserted that policy-makers and stakeholders require several types of reviews to inform the variety of policy-making processes they undertake (Lavis, 2009). Reviews of observational studies, qualitative studies, effectiveness studies, and economic evaluations can provide useful information for addressing the definition of a policy problem, identifying and exploiting windows of policy opportunity, and informing the development of monitoring and evaluation plans.

Health policy and program developers also need reviews that can inform interventions that address, among other things, social determinants of health (Bambra et al., 2010). There are two key research challenges related to identifying and implementing these types of interventions. First, evidence of the *causal links between social determinants and health outcomes* is limited. For example, descriptive epidemiological studies can highlight associations, but are not sufficient to identify the "effect levers" or key mechanisms of particular interventions (i.e., what makes the intervention work). Epidemiological studies can answer the "what" (the size of the effect) but not the "how" or "why" questions. Second, there is a lack of evidence of the effectiveness of *upstream* interventions—that is, interventions focused on changing institutional and social structures, rather than simply individual behaviours.

These challenges have been highlighted by Bambra and colleagues (2010) in their study of the twenty-first century "state of the systematic review evidence base" in developed countries that examined the effects of upstream health interventions on health outcomes and health inequalities. Notably, they found *no* systematic reviews on interventions that relate to macroeconomic, cultural, or environmental conditions aimed at reducing inequalities in human rights, income, and labour markets or controlling environmental hazards. Bambra and colleagues speculated that the void in systematic reviews of these types "may be as a result of our focus on intervention studies and it may well be that the evidence base therefore needs to be widened to include reviews of comparative (non-intervention) studies such as those conducted within social epidemiology" (2010, 13). They concluded that the public health systematic review evidence base on how to address social determinants of health is weak, and "does not yet allow us to say with any confidence what the effects of interventions on reducing health inequalities are, because differential impacts by socioeconomic position are rarely assessed" (Bambra et al., 2010, 15). We would add that the assessment of differential effects by social determinants of health such as gender, racialization, indigeneity, language of origin, dis/ability, sexual orientation, immigration/citizenship status, and others are even more rare.

Most interventions designed to address social determinants of health are complex, and establishing causal links between interventions and outcomes is often difficult. Mindful of these challenges, the Canadian Institute for Health Information Canadian Population Health Initiative (CIHI-CPHI) and the Canadian

Institutes of Health Research Institute of Population and Public Health (CIHR-IPPH) have noted that population health interventions "can include policy, program, and resource-distribution approaches. Their complexity arises from the fact that they are frequently aimed at more than one system level, may involve the use of multiple strategies, and can require implementation both within and outside the health sector. In addition, population health interventions are introduced into systems that are in and of themselves dynamic and complex" (CIHR-IPPH & CIHI-CPHI, 2010). Interventions within the health system—such as strategies to control or shorten wait times—pose similar challenges for evidence synthesis and assessment as interventions focused on other determinants of health.

We begin to address those challenges by examining, with a particular focus on gender and women's lives, the capacity of dominant systematic review methods to examine the sex and gender implications of wait times for hip- and knee-replacement surgeries. In the sections that follow, we describe how we applied these methods to assess their ability to provide sufficient evidence for a sex- and gender-based analysis.

## The Example of Wait Times

Wait times are a type of health system performance indicator. In the past, wait times were often difficult to measure because there was limited infrastructure for tracking patients' progress through the system, individual practitioners often kept their own lists and had different approaches to monitoring and tracking patients on those lists, and wait times were frequently not shared between practitioners, institutions, or provinces in Canada (Health Council of Canada, 2005). However, in 2004 the federal, provincial, and territorial first ministers in Canada (i.e., the premiers of the provinces and territories, and the prime minister of Canada) approved a *Ten Year Action Plan to Strengthen Health Care*, a response to widespread public concerns about access, timeliness, and account-ability in Canada's health care systems. To address these concerns, the plan included:

- a Wait Time Reduction Fund;
- objectives of better management and measurable reduc-tions of wait times in five priority areas (cancer, car-diac, diagnostic imaging, joint replacements, and sight restoration);
- the appointment of a federal advisor on wait times (Dr. Brian Postl).

In a separate but related event, in June 2005 the Supreme Court of Canada made its decision on the Chaoulli-Zeliotis case, rul-ing that the Government of Quebec could not prevent the sale of private insurance for health care procedures covered under the provincial public health insurance plan. The ruling stated that some health care wait times are unreasonably long and violate the rights of individual Canadians. As the federal advisor on wait times noted, "Public interest in the wait time issue and the need for government progress for a solution relating to issues of access increased as a result of this decision. It brought timeliness into the definition of access in a way that was new to the Canadian health care scene" (Postl, 2006, 17).

In 2005, Women and Health Care Reform was invited by the federal advisor on wait times to contribute to his report on wait times in the Canadian health care system. We authored a discus-sion paper entitled "New Questions, New Knowledge" (Jackson, Pederson & Boscoe, 2006) in which we applied sex- and gender-based analysis to the priority area of hip and knee replacements (also known as total joint arthroplasty, or TJA).[1] Given the time and resources available, we undertook a narrative review of the published literature and key items in the grey literature, comple-mented by a small number of key informant interviews. The first thing we learned was that provincial reports and websites on wait times did not reveal the gender of who was waiting for surgery because the wait times data were all reported in aggregate. Data were provided for "patients" in general or for those over or under age 65, but not for "women" and "men." We also found that the definition of wait time used in Canada was the time between when a specialist books the surgery and when the patient receives the surgery; this way of defining and measuring wait time excludes significant portions of the "patient journey" through the health care system and thus excludes significant elements of the waiting experience. Moreover, the literature includes very little information about how women and men are affected by waiting, which takes into account the kinds of paid/unpaid work they do, the supports they have, or their responsibilities as wage earners and/ or caregivers for family members and others. Further, when we examined surgery for hip and knee replacement, we found that most literature and available evidence on wait times for TJA did not address men's and women's differential prevalence of underlying conditions, nor the processes involved in being referred for surgery.

Yet there are significant differences between women and men in the prevalence of osteoarthritis (the condition underlying most referrals for TJA) as well as in how they utilize joint-replacement surgery. Specifically, women have twice the rate of osteoarthritis that men do, and both women and men "underutilize" surgery (i.e., they don't get it when they need it), but women underuse surgery three times more than men (Hawker et al., 2000). In our analysis we looked at three main areas to account for this difference in use. First, we looked at how women and men are diagnosed by health care providers as being in need of joint replacement. Second, we examined literature on how women and men report symptoms relevant to assessing the need for joint-replacement surgery and how clinicians make treatment decisions. Third, we looked at how patients themselves make decisions about treatment, particularly TJA.

We found that there is substantial evidence to suggest that

doctors make more errors in diagnosis and choose less aggressive treatment options for women than for men. For example, women report more severe pain levels, report pain more frequently, and report longer duration of pain than men, but women are less likely to receive treatment for it (Elderkin-Thompson & Waitzkin, 1999; Hoffman & Tarzian, 2001). Moreover, a majority of studies suggest there are racial and ethnic disparities in treatment for pain; specifically, across a range of health care settings, African-American and Hispanic patients are less likely than Whites to receive effective pain treatment (Bonham, 2001).

We also noted that some studies found that women were more likely than men to seek treatment for arthritis, but women with a potential need for hip or knee replacement were less likely than men to say they had discussed the procedure with a doctor. That is, although women seek treatment, surgery is not always raised as an option even when women are appropriate candidates. Surgery may be discussed less often for women patients for a variety of reasons. Physicians may hold beliefs about the risks of, indications for, and expected outcomes of TJA that make them consider women less appropriate candidates than men for the surgery and hence not discuss it with women as often (Hawker et al., 2000). For example, because women are less likely than men to be in the paid workforce, surgeons may perceive surgery to be less urgent for women than for men. Alternatively, women may be seen as less suitable candidates because they have less access to paid and unpaid help post-surgery to manage their recovery. Consequently, women are less likely than men to be referred to a specialist, or are referred to a surgeon after a longer period.

Finally, patients' concerns about lack of support after surgery may increase their unwillingness to undergo TJA and hence affect their decisions about surgery (Clark et al., 2004). Because elderly women are more likely to live alone than elderly men, it is reasonable to assume that women may have more difficulty getting support. In addition, because women are more likely than men to be caregivers for others, women may already be *providing* support, rather than receiving it, and this may affect their willingness to undergo surgery. Together, from these three lines of argument in the literature, we came to understand that more women than men were "waiting to wait" and that if they were not being referred for surgery by specialists, they were not reaching the wait list to be counted.

## From Narrative to Systematic Review

Our narrative review sensitized us to women's and men's divergent "patient journeys" through the health care system and the impact on their experiences of waiting for health care. We thus became focused on the need to address gender in primary and secondary research, knowledge synthesis, public debate, and policy-making on timely access to care. Mindful of the pervasiveness of the discourse of evidence-based medicine and its offspring, evidence-based/informed decision-making, we also wanted to explore and test mainstream methods for the production and synthesis of evidence to inform policy. Accordingly, we sought to develop a systematic review of the literature on TJA from a gender perspective, and in so doing, validate our initial narrative review. This process would also enable us to assess to what extent an SGBA could be undertaken using conventional methods. Based on this review, we hoped to make recommendations for strengthening the equity analysis potential of systematic review methods.

The purpose of our second review was *not* to assess the effectiveness of an intervention—a standard rationale for conducting a systematic review—but rather to examine how the literature represented the issue of wait times for TJA and, more specifically, whether sex and gender would be identified (alone or in association with other dimensions of social location such as age, race, and socio-economic status) as factors that influence wait times. Although our intended purpose differed from that of a conventional systematic review, our methods closely followed the standards outlined by the international Cochrane and Campbell collaborations and the National Institute for Clinical Excellence (NICE) in the UK.[2] Accordingly, we:

- identified research questions;
- established inclusion and exclusion criteria for studies;
- conducted a systematic library search of medical and social science databases to identify relevant literatures;
- critically reviewed the literature using multiple reviewers with a standardized format; and
- summarized our findings.

We posed three related research questions: What were the factors associated with wait times for total joint arthroplasty? Are sex and gender considered in this literature? If they were, what does the literature say about the influence of sex and gender on wait times for TJA?

While we identified a vast literature related to the topic of joint replacement, only a small portion of it explicitly addressed extra-clinical or contextual factors associated with waiting. We concluded that the dominant systematic review methodology and paradigm was not able to replicate the SGBA we had been able to produce using a narrative method. We believe this is because this review approach was designed to focus on clinical interventions ("finite" treatments); has a low tolerance for non-randomized controlled trials (RCT) evidence; and has limited ability to assess the effectiveness of complex interventions in complex social contexts (Bambra et al., 2010; Shepperd et al., 2009).

In fact, conventional systematic reviews are designed to strip context away—to standardize an intervention in order to isolate the factor that makes it "work." This is not a fatal critique of the Cochrane method applied to questions to which it is well suited, particularly experimental or quasi-experimental questions in tightly controlled conditions. As Popay notes, "The best developed approaches to systematic review are single issue-focused and designed to include a narrow range of evidence types" (2006, 107). However, the questions that guide evidence reviews in social determinants of health, sex- and gender-based analysis, and the evaluation of social policies and programs require methods that deal well with complexity and diverse kinds of evidence (Popay, 2006). This is where Cochrane-style systematic review methods may be applied, in error, beyond their scope.

# Assessing Complex Interventions Using a Realist Review

We understand wait times policies, strategies, measurement systems, and protocols are complex interventions. McCormack and colleagues contend that complex interventions are "comprised of theories, involve the actions of people, consist of a chain of steps or processes that interact and are rarely linear, are embedded in social systems, are prone to modification and exist in open systems that change through learning" (McCormack et al., 2006, 15). These policies, strategies, systems, and protocols are invested with power, and their construction and implementation privileges some groups over others. Our work on gender, wait times, and TJA has demonstrated that the complexity of these issues, or indeed of any intervention to address them, cannot be captured by a conventional Cochrane-style systematic review. On the other hand, a "realist review" approach, with its focus on complex interventions and careful attention to the contexts and processes in/through which they are implemented, may be able to rise to this challenge (Pawson, Greenhalgh, Harvey & Walshe, 2005).

Realist review is an approach to evidence synthesis that is sensitive to the complexities of modern health systems and is compatible with a multi-method, multidisciplinary evidence base. In contrast to other forms of knowledge synthesis, realist review focuses on the underlying "theories" of social interventions — that is, their mechanisms of action. Reviewers identify key steps in the chain of action in an intervention and examine the theories that explain those phases of the intervention. The realist review approach illuminates how combinations of individuals, relationships, institutions, and infrastructures in and through which an intervention is delivered affect how an intervention operates. The realist review is also sympathetic to the *in vivo* implementation of interventions—that is, how in "real-world" applications, interventions rarely unfold in a linear sequence as they tend to be modified through the negotiation and learning of various actors throughout the life of the intervention (Pawson et al., 2004, 2005; Shepperd et al., 2009).

In short, the realist review approach explicitly acknowledges that different contexts have an influence on how interventions work. Consequently, the focus is not only on *if* an intervention works, but *how, why, for whom,* and *in what circumstances* it works—in other words, the situated nature (the context) of interventions is key to their assessment, not something to be eliminated from the assessment process (Pawson et al., 2004, 2005; Shepperd et al., 2009). A realist review permits us to examine the particularities of a given context and to ask different questions about it. This can include questions about how a mechanism or intervention is gendered (and raced, classed, etc.). In contrast to conventional systematic reviews, realist reviews do not purport to generate generalizable findings that apply regardless of the context. Rather, realist reviews have a more modest goal, namely, to generate insights and potential theories about why something works in a particular circumstance. Realist reviews thus generate knowledge from particular conditions and it is the analyst's role to identify the ways that a given case might have general lessons to offer, including lessons about how gender and intersecting social locations shape experience, practice, and policy.

# Conclusion

With the range of techniques now available for evidence review and synthesis, it is imperative for researchers, clinicians, and policy actors to reflect critically upon those methods and ensure that the technique applied is suited to the research question(s) that drive(s) the review. It is also imperative to consider the extent to which a sex- and gender-based analysis (or other equity analysis) can be applied in the conduct of systematic reviews, as reviews that do not consider evidence relevant to equity risk missing key elements that should be taken into account in clinical and policy decision-making.

In this chapter, we have focused on the capacity of narrative and conventional Cochrane-style systematic review methods to capture the impact of sex and gender on wait times for total joint arthroplasty. We asked several foundational questions of the available evidence, including how "wait time" is defined, how the need for surgery is assessed, how valid measurement tools are for women and men across different social locations, and how women and men differ in terms of the contexts in which they seek (or do not seek) surgery (such as gendered social roles like caregiving or employment). We found that the complexity of these issues, or indeed of any intervention to address them, cannot be captured by a conventional Cochrane-style systematic review. In contrast, realist review, with its focus on complex interventions and careful attention to the contexts and processes in and through which they are implemented, appears to be a more appropriate and useful instrument for this type of assessment.

To properly address equity concerns, systematic review methods must be applied with the intention to assess equity across sex, gender, and the myriad of other social locations across which power, privilege, and resources are distributed. Sandra Harding (1989) famously asked the question "Is there a feminist method?" She answered, "Many of the most powerful examples of feminist research direct us to [...] place the researcher in the same critical plane as the overt subject matter, thereby recovering for scrutiny in the results of research the entire research process" (Harding, 1989, 29). Accordingly, any application of systematic review methods must be guided by the same commitments, reflexivity, and critical questions that have always guided Women and Health Care Reform's work: Why is this an issue for women? What are the issues for women? Which women? And what does this mean for women as patients, providers, and decision-makers?

## Notes

1. For a more detailed account of this narrative review, see Jackson, Pederson, and Boscoe (2009).
2. For additional information on systematic review methods, see the Cochrane Collaboration at http://www.cochrane-handbook.org; the National Institute for Health and Clinical Excellence at http://www.nice.org.uk; the Campbell Collaboration at http://www.campbellcollaboration.org.

## References

Bambra, C. (2009). Real world reviews: A beginner's guide to undertaking systematic reviews of public health policy interventions. *Journal of Epidemiology and Community Health* 1–15. Retrieved from http://www.ncbi.nlm.nih.gov/pubmed/19710043

Bambra, C., Gibson, M., Sowden, A., Wright, K., Whitehead, M. & Pettigrew, M. (2010). Tackling the wider social determinants of health and health inequalities: Evidence from systematic reviews. *Journal of Epidemiology and Community Health* 64(4), 284–291.

Bonham, V.I. (2001). Race, ethnicity, and pain treatment: Striving to understand the causes and solutions to the disparities in pain treatment. *Journal of Law, Medicine, and Ethics* 29(1), 52–68.

Boscoe, M., Tudiver, S., Doull, M. & Runnels, V.E. (2009). Sex and gender in systematic reviews. In B. Clow, A. Pederson, M. Haworth-Brockman & J. Bernier (Eds.), *Rising to the challenge: Sex- and gender-based analysis for health planning, policy, and research in Canada* (pp. 44–49). Halifax: Atlantic Centre of Excellence for Women's Health.

Canadian Institute for Health Information Canadian Population Health Initiative (CIHI-CPHI) & the Canadian Institute of Health

Research Institute of Population and Public Health (CIHR-IPPH). (2010). *Call for case abstracts for a new publication: Population health intervention research casebook.* Retrieved from http://www.cihr. ca/e/41599.html

Centre for Reviews and Dissemination. (2009). *Systematic reviews: CRD's guidance for undertaking reviews in health care.* Heslington: CRD.

Clark, J.P., Hudak, P.L., Hawker, G.A., Coyte, P.C., Mahomed, N.N., Kreeder, H.J. & Wright, J.G. (2004). The moving target: A qualitative study of elderly patients' decision-making regarding total joint replacement surgery. *Journal of Bone and Joint Surgery 86*(7), 1366–1374.

Dixon-Woods, M., Agarwal, S., Jones, D., Young, B. & Sutton, A. (2005). Synthesising qualitative and quantitative evidence: A review of possible methods. *Journal of Health Services Research and Policy 10*(1), 45–53.

Dixon-Woods, M., Cavers, D., Agarwal, S., Annandale, E., Arthur, A., Harvey, J., Hsu, R., Katbamna, S., Olsen, R., Smith, L., Riley, R. & Sutton, A.J. (2006). Conducting a critical interpretive synthesis of the literature on access to healthcare by vulnerable groups. *BMC Medical Research Methodology 6*(35), doi: 10.1186/1471-2288-6-35.

Elderkin-Thompson, V. & Waitzkin, H. (1999). Differences in clinical communication by gender. *Journal of General Internal Medicine 14*, 112–121.

Greenhalgh, T., Kristjansson, E. & Robinson V. (2007). Realist review to understand the efficacy of school feeding programmes. *British Medical Journal 335*, 858–861.

Harding S. (1989). Is there a feminist method? In N. Tuana (Ed.), *Feminism and science* (pp. 17–32). Bloomington: Indiana University Press.

Hawker, G.A., Wright, J.G., Coyte, P.C., Williams, J.I., Harvey, B., Glazier, R. & Bradley, E.M. (2000). Differences between men and women in the rate of use of hip and knee arthroplasty. *New England Journal of Medicine 342*(14), 1016–1021.

Health Council of Canada. (2005). *Health care renewal in Canada: Accelerating change.* Retrieved from http://www.healthcouncilcanada.ca/ docs/rpts/2005/Accelerating_Change_HCC_2005.pdf

Higgins, P.T. & Green, S. (2008*). Cochrane handbook for systematic* *reviews of interventions.* Version 5.0.1. The Cochrane Collaboration. Retrieved from http://www.cochrane-handbook.org

Hoffman, D.E. & Tarzian, A.J. (2001). The girl who cried pain: A bias against women in the treatment of pain. *Journal of Law, Medicine, and Ethics 29*(1), 13–27.

Jackson, B.E., Pederson, A. & Boscoe, M. (2006*). Gender-based analysis and wait times: New questions, new knowledge.* Toronto: Women and Health Care Reform. Retrieved from http://www.womenand-healthcarereform.ca/publications/genderwaittimesen.pdf

Jackson, B.E., A. Pederson, and M. Boscoe. (2009) Waiting to Wait: Improving Wait Times Evidence through Gender-Based Analysis. In Armstrong and Deadman (Eds.), *Women's Health: Intersections of Policy, Research and Practice* (pp 35-51). Toronto: Canadian Scholars Press.

Lavis, J.N. (2009). How can we support the use of systematic reviews in policymaking? *PLoS Medicine 6*(11).

Mays, N., Pope, C. & Popay, J. (2005). Systematically reviewing qualitative and quantitative evidence to inform management and policymaking in the health field. *Journal of Health Services Research and Policy 10*(Suppl. 1), 6–20.

Mays, N., Roberts, E. & Popay, J. (2001). Synthesising research evidence. In N. Fullop, P. Allen, A. Clarke & N. Black (Eds.), *Studying the organisation and delivery of health services: Research methods* (pp. 188–220). London: Routledge.

McCormack, B., Dewar, B., Wright, J., Garbett, R., Harvey, G. & Ballantine, K. (2006). *A realist synthesis of evidence relating to practice development: Final report to NHS Education for Scotland and NHS Quality Improvement Scotland.* Retrieved from http://www.nes.scot.nhs.uk/documents/publications/classa/finalreport4.pdf

Pawson, R., Greenhalgh, T., Harvey, G. & Walshe, K. (2004). *Realist synthesis: An introduction.* ESRC Research Methods Programme Working Paper Series, RMP Methods Paper 2/2004. Manchester: University of Manchester. Retrieved from http://www.ccsr.ac.uk/methods/publications/RMPmethods2.pdf

Pawson, R., Greenhalgh, T., Harvey, G. & Walshe, K. (2005). Realist review—a new method of systematic review designed for complex policy interventions. *Journal of Health Services Research and Policy* *10*(1), S1–S21.

Popay, J. (Ed.). (2006). *Moving beyond effectiveness in evidence synthesis: Methodological issues in the synthesis of diverse sources of evidence.* London: National Institute for Health and Clinical Excellence. Retrieved from http://www.nice.org.uk/niceMedia/docs/Moving_beyond_effectiveness_in_evidence_synthesis2.pdf

Popay, J. & Roberts, H. (2006). Introduction: Methodological issues in the synthesis of diverse sources of evidence. In J. Popay (Ed.), *Moving beyond effectiveness in evidence synthesis: Methodological issues in the synthesis of diverse sources of evidence.* London: National Institute for Health and Clinical Excellence.

Pope, C., Mays, N. & Popay, J., (2007). *Synthesising qualitative and quantitative health evidence: A guide to methods.* Maidenhead:Open University Press.

Postl, B.D. (2006). *Final report of the federal advisor on wait times.* Ottawa: Health Canada. Retrieved from http://www.hc-sc.gc.ca/hcs-sss/alt_formats/hpb-dgps/pdf/pubs/2006-wait-attente/index-eng.pdf

Sandelowski, M., Docherty, S. & Emden, C. (1997). Qualitative metasynthesis: Issues and techniques. *Research in Nursing and Health 20,* 365–371.

Shepperd, S., Lewin, S., Straus, S., Clarke, M., Eccles, M.P., Fitzpatrick, R., Wong, G. & Sheikh, A. (2009). Can we systematically review studies that evaluate complex interventions? *PLoS Medicine* 6(8).

van der Knaap, L.M., Leeuw, F.L., Bogaerts, S. & Nijssen, L.T.J. (2008). Combining Campbell standards and the realist evaluation approach: The best of two worlds? *American Journal of Evaluation* *29*(1), 48–57.

# CHAPTER 4
# Maternity Care

MARGARET HAWORTH-BROCKMAN, BARBARA CLOW,
AND RACHEL RAPAPORT BECK

## Introduction

For many years Women and Health Care Reform deliberately
avoided working on women's sexual and reproductive health.
Women's health is often reduced to sexual and reproductive
health and we wanted to move beyond this traditional definition to a consideration of other aspects of women's well-being.
Nevertheless, childbirth is the leading reason women seek health
care in Canada, and maternity care, like health care in general,
has been subject to extensive reforms that have implications for
women receiving and providing care. We approached the analysis of maternity care reforms with our usual questions: Why is
this a women's issue? What are the issues for women? Which
women are most affected? While the answers to these questions
might seem obvious since child-bearing is specific to women,
it is important to bear in mind that gender as well as sex influences reproductive experiences. Pregnancy, labour, breastfeeding,
and postnatal care—even contraception and conception—are all
affected by gender norms and expectations. Furthermore, women

who receive and provide maternity care are not a uniform group, and the effects of reforms have different implications for different women as providers and as those with maternity care needs.

Members of Women and Health Care Reform have individually pursued research and policy work related to maternity care, generating new knowledge as well as providing information and insight about trends and developments internationally, nationally, provincially, and locally. In 2006, the group collectively turned its attention to the implications of reforms to maternity care for those giving and receiving services, and the following year published a plain-language analysis (WHCR, 2007). In 2008, we co-hosted a workshop on Environments and Maternal Health, and commissioned a background paper to analyze the gender dimensions of the social, clinical, and work environments of maternity care in Canada (Sutherns, 2008). This chapter provides an overview of what we learned about maternity care reforms, an analysis of more recent reforms to maternity care, and the implications of these changes for women.

The phrase "maternity care" means different things to different people. For some, the term encompasses care only during pregnancy and labour, while for others it applies to a range of services that women need before, during, and after a baby is born. In this chapter we consider maternity care to be health care sought and provided in the 12 months that span pregnancy, delivery, and the weeks following birth—the child-bearing year. We stress that the child-bearing year should not be regarded as separate from the rest of women's lives, and that getting pregnant, staying pregnant, giving birth, and providing care to an infant are all very different experiences for individual women. Women's experiences and needs are complex and diverse. They include dealing with the challenges of infertility, pursuing adoption or other ways to bring children into families, planning or not planning to conceive, terminating unwanted pregnancies, seeking specific kinds of care during pregnancy and finding it (or not), choosing whether or not to breastfeed, and a host of personal considerations that arise before, during, and after pregnancy. All of these experiences are gendered and must be understood in relation to the norms, roles, and expectations attached to being female and having a baby.

We start with a reflection on the factors we described in 2008 that were creating a "new normal" in maternity care. Whereas "normal" used to refer to pregnancies and births that were uncomplicated and had few or no interventions, we found that the environments around the child-bearing year were fundamentally changing maternity care. From there we look at more recent developments and what lies ahead.

## Shifts to a "New Normal"

In our review of the environments of birth and health care reforms related to maternity care, we found a variety of factors that contribute to a "new normal." The shift was not entirely by design, but rather was a convergence of changes in health human resources, in skill sets, in how and where maternity care is provided, as well as in social and cultural trends. Fewer practitioners are available and fewer facilities are equipped or open for the provision of maternity care. Women and their health care providers are also increasingly nervous about labour and delivery while rates of medical intervention, such as induced and augmented labour, Caesarean section, and epidural anaesthesia are climbing. These changing perspectives affect what normal maternity care and childbirth mean.

### HEALTH OUTCOMES FOR WOMEN AND NEWBORNS

As early as 2002, the Organisation for Economic Co-operation and Development (OECD) reported that maternal and newborn health in Canada were deteriorating, with Canada's international ranking declining on several key indicators. Compared with 10 years earlier, Canada's ranking for rates of infant mortality had plunged from sixth to twenty-first, while our ranking for maternal mortality slipped from second to eleventh (cited in SOGC, 2008, 6). While these trends were evident for the Canadian population as a whole, it was also becoming clear that Aboriginal women (Inuit, First Nations, and Métis) were particularly at risk of having complications during birth as well as higher rates of maternal morbidity and mortality. Important gains in maternal and newborn health that had been achieved through public health measures, better nutrition, and access to services were clearly being lost. Evidence suggests that the worsening of maternal and infant health outcomes is linked to rising rates of medical and surgical interventions during labour and delivery, and possibly to the loss of local birthing assistance or facilities for women who live outside of the larger cities and towns in Canada (Kornelsen & Gryzbowski, 2005a, 2005b).

MATERNITY CARE PROVIDERS

Changes in health human resources in recent years have clearly affected the type and quality of care available to women in the child-bearing year. Through the middle years of the twentieth century family physicians were the most likely attendants at births (CIHI, 2004). A shift to the more specialized care of obstetricians became pronounced in the 1980s and the 1990s as family physicians became less likely to provide on-call services for pregnant women (SOGC, 2008). Health care reforms were responsible, at least in part, for this shift. Hospital and maternity ward closures (particularly in rural Canada), which were designed to cut costs and reduce duplication, resulted in cuts to nurses, beds, and other resources for maternity care, making it more difficult or even impossible for family doctors to deliver babies in hospitals. In some jurisdictions there were stricter guidelines for the local availability and capability for Caesarean sections (CIHI, 2004; Kornelsen & Gryzbowski, 2005b).[1] At the same time, by the end of the 1990s Canadian obstetricians as a group were getting older, with few younger physicians moving into the specialty (Sutherns, 2008; SOGC, 2008). However, in the early 1990s the social movement to reinstate midwives as primary providers for women through pregnancy, birth, and the early postpartum period succeeded, with legislation and public policy to regulate the profession introduced in some provinces. Re-establishing midwifery was an important, perhaps even critical, reform, which helped to alleviate some of the pressure on maternity care. Yet midwifery remained unavailable in some parts of the country and was developing slowly in most provinces (Sutherns, 2008). Moreover, the changing profile of maternity care providers was not evenly coordinated despite the fact that efficient referral and backup are essential as no one can be on call for women in labour around the clock indefinitely.

## MEDICALIZATION

Much has been written about the medicalization of pregnancy and birth (Klein, 2004; Green & Baston, 2007; Block, 2007) and it is difficult to disentangle the various reasons for the increasing use of interventions during labour and delivery (Enkin, 2006). Certainly women have long been interested in pain relief, requesting and using both anaesthetics and analgesics (Van Wagner, 2008). But the merits of medicinal pain relief remain unclear. For example, epidural anaesthetics are a popular choice for women and their providers (O'Brien, Young & Chalmers 2009), but there has been consistent evidence that epidurals do not improve health outcomes for infants or mothers and, more importantly, that one intervention in labour, like the use of an epidural or elective induction, leads to more interventions (Anim-Somuah, Smyth & Howell, 2005; Dunne et al., 2009). Research trials have found that pain can be well managed — in most cases — when personal, one-to-one care is available throughout labour (McGrath & Kennell, 2008). Unfortunately, the pressures on maternity care providers and facilities created by health care reforms means that this labour-intensive approach to pain management is often not available.

Similar trends can be tracked for other types of interventions, such as Caesarean section. In a survey of close to 3,000 maternity care providers in Canada, Klein et al. found that 20 percent of obstetricians believed that Caesarean section was safer than vaginal birth and another 20 percent felt that it was at least as safe as vaginal birth (Klein et al., 2009). While providers describe the medical merits of intervention, they are also influenced by a desire for greater control over birth. Klein et al. (2009) found that approximately 7 percent of obstetricians would themselves choose Caesarean section because it would alleviate the unpredictability of birthing. For providers, and possibly for the health care system in general, active management of labour and birth is preferable to waiting with a woman through the unknown.

### A CULTURE OF FEAR

Increasing rates of intervention also point to a growing culture of fear surrounding childbirth among providers as well as among women. Women's fears of childbirth—of pain, injury, and potentially death—persist for a number of reasons. Stories shared among women and between generations, as well as media representations of birthing fuel fear and, as Van Wagner (2008) has observed, there are few public education campaigns to counter frightening stories and images of birth. But Sutherns (2008) also found that physicians, nurses, and other providers and administrators have come to view childbirth as "a dangerous event to be feared" (p. 17). Indeed, she noted that, "If (providers) see birth as a series of potential misadventures, their counsel to their patients cannot help but be affected" (Sutherns, 2008, 17). Certainly there is evidence to suggest that women increasingly perceive Caesarean sections as low risk and vaginal births as dangerous, despite considerable evidence to the contrary (Weaver, Stratham & Richards, 2007).[2] At the same time, while infant deaths are devastating for mothers and families, they have also become a professional and a health care system liability. As Jennifer Block (2007) writes, "[e]verything possible is done" to manage care and to show that care has been well managed, always with the worry of litigation in mind (p. 43).

While these kinds of beliefs and preferences might be understandable, particularly in the absence of public and professional education, they are also redefining a healthy, "normal" birth as one that includes significant intervention (SOGC, 2008), which does not match evidence-based professional guidelines (WHO 2006, Health Canada 2000).[3] Hospital systems that have adopted highly medical responses to women in labour have not demonstrated an ability to change routines to the fewer interventions recommended by research.

## INFORMATION GAPS

Appropriate and sustainable reforms of maternity care require reliable information, but maternity care is not tracked consistently across Canada. We do not, for example, have comprehensive information about obstetricians and family physicians providing intrapartum and postpartum care; the numbers of midwives caring for women at different stages in the child-bearing year; the supply of labour and delivery or public health nurses for women in the child-bearing year; the outcomes of midwifery-attended births; or comparisons of infant and maternal outcomes under different models of maternity care. We also have limited information about the needs and experiences of diverse groups of women. For example, a 2010 study in Winnipeg found that a substantial proportion (up to 21 percent) of inner-city women were not seeking or receiving prenatal care, but further research is needed to understand if this is a choice women make or if they cannot get the care they want (Heaman, 2010). These information gaps make it difficult to assess where reforms are taking place and how they affect both the women who receive care and those whose job it is to give care.

## POLICIES AND STANDARDS

Sutherns (2008) described efforts to improve maternity care through practice standards based on research evidence and by encouraging providers to work collaboratively in the interests of women-centred care. A large-scale project of the Society for Obstetricians and Gynecologists, the Multidisciplinary Collaborative

Primary Maternity Care Project (or MCP[2]), provided recommendations for collaborative, collegial models of practice. By the time MCP[2] drew to a close in 2008 the project had generated dozens of reports, presentations, and guidelines, as well as key recommendations for maternity care reform. The collaborative models of practice promoted by MCP[2] partners were suggested to be the best means to improve health outcomes for mothers and babies while addressing the crisis of declining numbers of maternity care providers. Unfortunately, this vision for maternity care reform was not matched by national professional or political leadership and the resources necessary to effect change have been made available only piecemeal in some provinces.

Women and Health Care Reform has long maintained that maternity care is on the periphery of policy agendas because it is both ordinary—and therefore invisible—and extraordinarily difficult to "fix." Sutherns's (2008) review confirmed this interpretation. She argued that one of the most alarming aspects of changes in maternity care is that they are happening without deliberation and without drawing much attention: "We are on the verge of a 'new normal' for maternity care in Canada, one that is being driven in large part by health human resource shortages, changes in skill sets and cultural and social trends in the provision of care, rather than by deliberate design" (p. 1). But Sutherns's analysis also demonstrated that good maternity care exists in Canada, and that there is a genuine desire among providers to find new models for working together to keep women at the centre of care.

## The Shifts Continue

The latest research and policy literature on maternity care demonstrate both change and continuity, neither of which can be neatly categorized as beneficial or detrimental. Fertility rates are rising, as is the age of women giving birth for the first time. But rates of interventions continue to climb as well. Rural and northern women must travel farther for care and other vulnerable groups show worsening health outcomes. Midwifery is now more widely available, but maternity care providers remain scarce in many parts of the country. Taken together, change and continuity add up to an ongoing shift and even a crisis in maternity care in Canada.

## DEMOGRAPHICS

After many years of declining birth rates, the number of babies being born in Canada is increasing. According to Statistics Canada (2009), 3.7 percent more babies were born in 2007 than in 2006. While this may be a temporary trend, this is the fastest annual increase since 1989. At the same time, more women over the age of 35 are giving birth, many for the first time. In 2005, 11 percent of first births were for women over 35 years, a nearly threefold increase since 1987 (Statistics Canada, 2009). Women in their early thirties were also more likely to give birth for the first time, an increase from 15 percent in 1987 to 26 percent in 2005. By 2006, the highest fertility rate was among women in their early thirties (Statistics Canada, 2008). During the same period, fertility rates for teenage females have declined, except among young First Nations and Inuit women.

## HEALTH OUTCOMES

Shifting fertility trends are not necessarily correlated with significant changes in health outcomes. For example, a review by Statistics Canada (2008) found "no significant differences in health, behaviour and cognitive outcomes" among infants and children born to first-time mothers over the age of 35, and babies born to older mothers were "significantly more likely to have been breastfed and breastfed longer compared with children of mothers in the younger group."

There are some subpopulations of women and babies who continue to be at risk, however. For instance, while the proportion of low–birth weight babies (defined as under 2,500 g) in the First Nations population was lower than average—5.3 percent versus

6 percent for the general population—rates of high birth weight (above 4,000 g) among First Nations mothers were higher than average—21 percent compared to 13 percent among the non–First Nations population. Low birth weights and high birth weights both have potentially adverse outcomes (Human Resources and Development Canada, 2002). Low–birth weight babies are more likely to die in the first year of life and to experience developmental disabilities and disease. High birth weight is associated with increased maternal and infant risk for perinatal complications and adverse outcomes, such as birth injuries. A 2010 review of published literature found that the infant mortality rate for First Nations and off-reserve Status Indians between 1991 and 2000 was almost twice the "non–First Nations" infant mortality rate in Manitoba. The rate disparity was "most striking for the postneonatal period" (Smylie, Fell & Ohlsson, 2010, 147). Similarly, the infant mortality rate among Inuit residing in Quebec was more than four times the rate for francophone women in Quebec (Smylie, Fell & Ohlsson, 2010). Another 2010 study compared 13,000 births in Inuit-inhabited regions to 4 million births in other regions in Canada between 1990 and 2000. The study found "large and persistent disparities in fetal and infant mortality between Inuit-inhabited areas and other areas of Canada" (Luo et al., 2010, 238). The same study showed that the risks of preterm birth, stillbirth, and especially infant death were substantially elevated. The rate of infant death in the Inuit-inhabited regions of Canada was 16.5 per 1,000 live births during the study period, which almost equalled the rate in all of Canada in 1971 (Luo et al., 2010, 239).[4] Aboriginal infant mortality rates remain high regardless of geography (northern, isolated, or urban setting), but this is not true for non-Aboriginal infants (Luo et al., 2010). Since the infant mortality rate is in some cases tied to health services, these figures indicate that First Nations (and Inuit) women are not receiving adequate maternity care (Smylie, Fell & Ohlsson, 2010; Luo et al., 2010).

The health outcome data for First Nations and Inuit women are alarming, but there are many other subpopulations of women about whom we know very little. We do not, for instance, have equivalent data for Métis and non-Status Indians, for women with disabilities, for African-Canadian women, and many other subpopulations. Such gaps in knowledge, identified by Sutherns (2008) and others, continue to hamper efforts to remediate and provide the kinds of maternity care that women in Canada want and need.

Health outcomes are also affected by new conditions or by changing rates of certain conditions. As elsewhere in the world, in Canada there is an increasing proportion of people who are overweight or obese, including women in the child-bearing year. Maternal complications of overweight and obesity include infertility, hypertension, gestational diabetes, Caesarean delivery, and hemorrhage (Arendas, Qiu & Gruslin, 2008). Fetal complications of maternal overweight and obesity include fetal distress and death, stillbirth, increased birth weight, and congenital anomalies (Arendas, Qiu & Gruslin, 2008). Further, some research has linked maternal overweight and obesity with decreased rates of breastfeeding, which has health implications for both mother and child, including higher rates of childhood obesity (Amir & Donath, 2007). A Swedish study asked women about being pregnant and obese and found that obese pregnant women constituted a vulnerable population because both of their conditions are highly visible (Nyman et al., 2008). Many women felt guilt over the potential dangers that obesity posed for themselves and their unborn children, and many felt humiliated by their health care providers (Nyman et al., 2008). Canadian maternity care providers are working toward clinical guidelines for maternity care for women who are overweight and obese, and we hope that women's needs and concerns are at the centre of the care recommendations.

**MATERNITY CARE PROVIDERS**
It is difficult to get maternity care in some parts of Canada. Diminished interest among family doctors in providing intrapartum care and fewer doctors receiving specialist training both

contribute to the shortage of maternity care providers. The lack of role models has created a self-perpetuating cycle. Rowe (2008) notes that we may soon become desensitized to the crisis and the shortage of specialists in obstetrics and gynecology. He suggests a reversal of attitude and calls on his colleagues to demonstrate their "obvious passion" for obstetrics. He adds, "We must show hesitant trainees why they should want to be like us" (Rowe, 2008, 558).

Shortages or uneven distribution of maternity care providers mean that many women must travel to give birth if they live outside of the major cities and towns in Canada. The Canadian Institute of Health Information (2010) reports that "maternal and newborn stays accounted for almost one-quarter of out-of-province/territory hospitalizations" (p. 2), and that the majority of these admissions were planned. Pregnant women and newborns were hospitalized a median distance of 78 km from home, which in Canada means that some women are travelling much greater distances to receive maternity care. First Nations and Inuit are especially likely to have to leave home weeks before their babies are due. Kornelsen and Gryzbowski (2005a, 2005b) have documented some of the far-reaching effects of removing birth from small British Columbia communities, including increased costs, disconnection for entire communities, and poorer health outcomes for women and infants. They also found that the shift from family physicians to obstetricians providing intrapartum care, along with changing practice standards and hospital closures, were among the most significant factors forcing women to travel farther from home to give birth. In a sparsely populated country such as Canada, some women will likely always have to travel to receive care for birth, but the authors of the MCP$^2$ project (2006) and others have noted that moving to more innovative care models and making better use of nurses, midwives, and other providers can help women stay closer to home and family through pregnancy and labour.

### INTERVENTIONS DURING BIRTH

The 2008 Canadian Perinatal Health Report recorded continued rises in the number of medical and surgical interventions during labour and delivery, including inductions (p. 73), operative vaginal delivery (p. 82), and Caesarean sections (p. 77). A 2009 survey of mothers reported that 57.3 percent who delivered or attempted to deliver vaginally had an epidural or spinal anaesthetic, and more than 80 percent of these women found the medicinal pain relief helpful (PHAC, 2009). High rates of induction, epidural use, and Caesarean section are worrisome because research consistently demonstrates that these and other routinely used interventions lead to poorer outcomes for mothers and for babies. As in the past, it would seem that women and their providers may not be discussing the full range of birthing options. According to the same report, only 75 percent of women reported having information about pain management prior to giving birth (PHAC, 2009).

Romano and Lothian (2008, 96–100) make the following recommendations for obstetric nurses and other providers to help reduce the medicalization of birth:

- Allow labour to begin naturally, without intervention or induction.
- Give pregnant woman the freedom to move about during labour.
- Provide continuous one-to-one support during labour.
- Do not routinely use interventions in labour.
- Encourage spontaneous, unhurried pushing in the second stage in non-supine positions.
- Do not separate mothers and babies following birth.

These recommendations are consistent with more than 35 years of research, but it is not clear that they can or will change the culture of birth in Canada. Research evidence has not been translated widely into practice, in part because obstetric training may not include enough unmanaged births, and partly because change takes time that maternity care providers can ill afford. As Romano and Lothian (2008) note,

> In the current maternity care environment, providing evidence-based nursing care that promotes, protects, and supports normal birth is a challenge.... Modern obstetric units are well-equipped to deal with high-risk or complicated births, but the policies, protocols and physical infrastructure are not ideal for physiological birth. (p. 101)

The authors recommend that labour and delivery nurses are well placed to help women, hospitals, and the people who work in them to return to less technological and more respectful birth assistance. This would include taking time to help women (and nurses) become familiar with evidence-based changes, such as how to relieve pain in labour, so that they can make genuinely informed choices about their care.

As in the past, women and providers have many anxieties about childbirth. Klein et al. (2009, 2011) interviewed obstetricians in Canada to understand better why obstetrical practice remains focused on interventions and managed care rather than the more supportive care that evidence demonstrates is better for women and babies. Obstetricians under the age of 40, 80 percent of whom were women, spoke about the inherent dangers in childbirth. They were unwilling to consider vaginal births after Caesarean section, and they were generally uninterested in women's own plans for their births. In the authors' assessment, the obstetricians' surgical training is partly responsible for resistance to supportive non-interventionist care during labour (Klein et al., 2011). Similarly, women continue to harbour fears about childbirth, and many lack essential information that could help to allay fears and equip them to make decisions about their birthing experiences. In a series of interviews conducted throughout their pregnancies, Klein et al. (2009) spoke with 1,300 women who were having their first babies. Although women's knowledge about pregnancy and birth increased over the course of their three trimesters, fewer than 50 percent had enough information, in the authors' opinions, to give their informed consent for interventions at the time labour began. The Mothers' Experience Survey, conducted by the Public Health Agency of Canada (2009), appears to support these findings. The survey indicated that women with lower education and income levels were more likely to report interventions during labour, compared with women who had higher levels of education.

Are fears among providers and women driving the continued use of medical interventions in birth? Over 6,400 women across the country were interviewed about their experiences during pregnancy, labour, birth, and postpartum (PHAC, 2009). Women reported lying flat on their back for birth (47.9 percent and many in stirrups), being induced (44.8 percent), or having labour augmented with drugs (37.3 percent), and enduring shaving and enemas, as well as pushing on the abdomen, to speed delivery. While it is difficult to find definitive evidence linking fear and intervention, strong cultural and societal fears about birth do seem to be an important factor in the disconnection between the research evidence for few interventions and the routines and practices for increased management in pregnancy and birth that are so often used.

## STANDARDS AND POLICIES

The National Birthing Initiative, released in 2008 by the Society of Obstetricians and Gynecologists of Canada (SOGC, 2008), calls for action in seven areas.[5] One of the recommendations is for federal leadership to underwrite "a national body to oversee the planning, implementation and evaluation of long-term multidisciplinary collaborative care strategies for maternity care" (p. 3). Despite good intentions and a desire to invest in change demonstrated by professional organizations such as the SOGC, collaborative care models remain, for the most part, unrealized. MCP[2] produced solid recommendations for the reform of maternity care, but it is one of several instances in which people have been brought together and have developed consensus, but there has been no follow-up. Even the reintroduction of midwifery has not solved the crisis of maternity care because provincial regulation has been uneven, and care delivery models and payment systems to providers cannot easily accommodate the supportive approach to care that is at the heart of midwifery.

## Looking Ahead

Two and a half years after our review of maternity care in Canada, it feels as if some things are changing, but little is improving. Many women and providers continue to fear childbirth and prefer managed to supportive care. We still do not have enough maternity care providers to meet the needs of women across the country and we do not have enough information about subpopulations of women. New challenges are emerging, such as rising rates of overweight and obesity, as well as changing fertility rates and shifts in the age of first-time mothers.

But there are also important and beneficial reforms taking place. There are new models of shared practice and collaboration in some parts of Canada where maternity care is no longer in "crisis." Birth centres in northern Quebec, for instance, (and one planned for Winnipeg) provide maternity care close to women's homes, as well as training facilities for new midwives and other providers. Rising Caesarean section rates and other interventions in birth are worrisome, but they are not going unnoticed. Providers and women, together, are beginning to challenge the need for intervention. The Mothers' Experiences report demonstrates that women's experiences of child-bearing, indeed the entire child-bearing year, can be considered in the context of their lives, making maternity care holistic and integrated, rather than an isolated effort to manage labour and birth (PHAC, 2009).

Perhaps the biggest concern is the difficulty of keeping birth in the public eye and on political agendas. When the OECD released its most recent figures on infant and maternal mortality, and as international attention turned toward Canada in the weeks and months leading up to the G8/G20 summit in 2010, maternity care came into sharper focus. Maternal mortality is an international standard of basic public and population health. Countries with high maternal mortality rates are generally doing poorly overall, compared with countries with low maternal mortality. Consequently, the World Health Organization has identified the importance of basic supports, such as clean water, adequate food and sanitation, and skilled birth attendants, as critical resources to reduce maternal mortality and contribute to development (WHO, n.d.). The United Nations Millennium Development Goals likewise include reductions in maternal mortality (United Nations, 2000, Goal #5). While the Canadian government declared its intention to contribute to improved maternal and child health internationally, the state of maternity care, particularly the appalling statistics for Aboriginal women, received scant attention (Picard, 2010; Priest, 2010). This is a big problem. In countries such as Canada, where maternal mortality is generally low, the very ordinariness of childbirth (from a policy perspective) can keep it at the fringes of media, public, and policy attention. But as this discussion makes clear, inattention to maternity care is affecting women's health, and it is incumbent upon all of us to remind policy-makers, practitioners, and the public about the importance of maternity care as a women's issue. Moreover, we must continue to make sure that maternity care is understood in the context of women's lives, both as providers and recipients of care.

# Notes

1. In one part of Manitoba, local deliveries were stopped because there was no on-call pediatrician available, a requirement the hospital had instituted.
2. This same study found that very few women ask for a Caesarean section, but many physicians continue to believe that maternal request is the primary cause of increased Caesarean section rates (Weaver et al., 2007).
3. See, for example, the 2008 Canadian Perinatal Surveillance Report, which measures interventions, but not births without interventions.
4. The infant mortality rate for the rest of Canada at the time was 4.6 per 1,000 live births. Authors note that birth registrations have not been consistent, and this fact can affect earlier calculated rates of mortality and morbidity (Smylie, Fell & Ohllson, 2010; Luo et al., 2010).
5. See http://www.sogc.org/projects/pdf/BirthingStrategyVersionc-Jan2008.pdf for the seven recommendations.

# References

Amir, L.H. & Donath, S. (2007). A systematic review of maternal obesity and breastfeeding intention, initiation, and duration. *BMC Pregnancy Childbirth 7*, 9.

Anim-Somuah, M., Smyth, R. & Howell, C. (2005). Epidural versus non-epidural or no analgesia in labour. *Cochrane Database of Systematic Reviews 4*. Art. no.: CD000331 DOI: 10.1002/14651858.CD000331.pub2.

Arendas, A., Qiu, Q. & Gruslin, A. (2008). Obesity in pregnancy: Pre-conceptional to postpartum consequences. *Journal of Obstetrics and Gynaecology Canada 30*(6), 477–488.

Block, J. (2007). *Pushed: The painful truth about childbirth and modern maternity care*. Cambridge: De Capo Press.

Canadian Institute for Health Information (CIHI). (2004). *Giving birth in Canada: Providers of maternity and infant care.* Ottawa: Canadian Institute for Health Information.

Canadian Institute for Health Information (CIHI). (2010). *Have health card will travel: Out of province/territory patients.* Ottawa: Canadian Institute for Health Information.

Dunne, C., Da Silva, O., Schmidt, G. & Natale, R. (2009). Outcomes of elective labour induction and elective Cesarean section in low-risk pregnancies between 37 and 41 weeks' gestation. *Journal of Obstetrics and Gynaecology Canada 31*(12), 1124–1130.

Enkin, M. (2006). Beyond evidence: The complexity of maternity care (guest editorial). *Birth 33*(4), 254–271.

Green, J.M. & Baston, H.A. (2007). Have women become more willing to accept obstetric interventions and does this relate to mode of birth? Data from a prospective study. *Birth 34*(1), 6–13.

Health Canada. (2000). *Family centred maternity and newborn care: National guidelines.* Ottawa: Minister of Public Works and Government Services.

Heaman, M. (2010). *Factors associated with inadequate prenatal care among inner-city women in Winnipeg.* Summary of results for knowledge translation workshop, Winnipeg, May 6, 2010.

Human Resources and Development Canada. (2002). *Well-being of Canada's young children: Government of Canada report.* http://www. socialunion.gc.ca/ecd/2002/reportb-e.pdf.

Klein, M.C. (2004). Quick fix culture: The Caesarean section-on-demand debate. *Birth 32*(3), 161–164.

Klein, M.C., Kaczorowski, J., Hall, W.A., Fraser, W., Listonn, R.M., Eftekhary, S., et al. (2009). The attitudes of Canadian maternity care practitioners towards labour and birth: Many differences but important similarities. *Journal of Obstetrics and Gynaecology Canada 31*(9), 827–840.

Klein, M.C., Liston, R., Fraser, W.D., Baradarn, N., Hearps, S.J.C., Tomkinson, J., et al. (2011). Attitudes of the new generation of Canadian obstetricians: How do they differ from the predecessors? *Birth 38*(2), 1–11.

Kornelsen, J. & Grzybowski, S. (2005a). The costs of separation: The birth experiences of women in isolated and remote communities in

British Columbia. *Canadian Women Studies Journal 24*, 75–80.

Kornelsen, J. & Grzybowski, S. (2005b). Is local maternity care an optional service in rural communities? *Journal of Obstetrics and Gynaecology of Canada 27*, 329–331.

Luo, Z.C., Senecal, S., Simonet, F., Guimond, E., Penney, C. & Wilkins, R. (2010). Birth outcomes in the Inuit-inhabited areas of Canada. *Canadian Medical Association Journal 182*(3), 235–242.

McGrath, S.K. & Kennell, J.H. (2008). A randomized controlled trial of continuous labour support for middle-class couples: Effect on Caesarean delivery rates. *Birth 35*(2), 92–97.

Multidisciplinary Collaborative Primary Maternity Care Project. Retrieved from http://www.mcp2.ca/

Nyman, V.M.K., Prebensen, A.K. & Gullvi, E.M. (2008). Obese women's experiences of encounters with midwives and physicians during pregnancy and childbirth. *Midwifery 26*(4), 424–429.

O'Brien, B., Young, D. & Chalmers, B. (2009). Pain management. In *What mothers say: The Canadian maternity experiences survey*. Ottawa: Public Health Agency of Canada.

Picard, A. (2010). Procedures for delivering babies vary markedly across Canada. *Globe and Mail*, May 18. Retrieved from http://www.theglobeandmail.com/life/health/procedures-for-delivering-babies-vary-markedly-across-canada/article1573472/

Priest, L. (2010). Canada's reputation for low infant mortality takes stunning decline. *Globe and Mail*, May 22. Retrieved from http://www.theglobeandmail.com/news/politics/canadas-reputation-for-low-infant-mortality-takes-stunning-decline/article1578103/

Public Health Agency of Canada. (2008). *Canadian Perinatal Health Report*, 2008 Edition. Retrieved from: http://www.phac-aspc.gc.ca/publicat/2008/cphr-rspc/pdf/cphr-rspc08-eng.pdf.

Public Health Agency of Canada (PHAC). (2009). *What mothers say: The Canadian maternity experiences survey*. Ottawa: Public Health Agency of Canada.

Romano, A.M. & Lothian, J.A. (2008). Promoting, protecting, and supporting normal birth: A look at the evidence. *Journal of Obstetric,*

*Gynecologic, and Neonatal Nursing 37*(1), 94–105.

Rowe, T. (2008). Crisis? What crisis? *Journal of Obstetrics and Gynaecology Canada 30*(7), 557–558.

Smylie, J., Fell, D. & Ohlsson, A., the Joint Working Group on First Nations, Indian, Inuit, and Métis Infant Mortality of the Canadian Perinatal Surveillance System. (2010). A review of Aboriginal infant mortality rates in Canada: Striking and persistent Aboriginal/non-Aboriginal inequities. *Canadian Journal of Public Health 101*(2), 143–148.

Society of Obstetricians and Gynecologists of Canada (SOGC). (2008). *A national birth initiative for Canada*. Ottawa: The Society of Obstetricians and Gynecologists of Canada.

Statistics Canada. (2008). Health and development of children of older first-time mothers. *The Daily*. Retrieved from http://www.statcan.gc.ca/daily-quotidien/080924/dq080924a-emg.htm

Statistics Canada. (2009). Births. *The Daily*. Retrieved from http://www.statcan.gc.ca/daily-quotidien/090922/dq090922b-eng.htm

Sutherns, R. (2008). *Human resources and the environment of birth in Canada: On the brink of a 'new normal'. Women and health care reform*. Retrieved from http://www.womenandhealthcarereform.ca

Tepper, J. (2004). *The evolving role of Canada's family physicians, 1992–2001*. Canadian Institute for Health Information. Retrieved from http://secure.cihi.ca/cihiweb/products/PhysiciansREPORT_eng.pdf

United Nations. (2000). *Millennium development goals — Goal #5*. Retrieved from http://www.un.org/millenniumgoals/maternal.shtml

Van Wagner, V. (2008). *Perceptions of birth: The challenge of public education and our popular and professional cultures*. Presented at British Columbia Cesarean Section Consensus Conference, January 24, 2008.

Weaver, J., Stratham, R. & Richards, M. (2007). Are there "unnecessary" Cesarean sections? Perceptions of women and obstetricians about Cesarean sections for nonclinical indications. *Birth 34*(1) (March), 32–41.

Women and Health Care Reform (WHCR). (2007). *Maternity matters*. Winnipeg: Women and Health Care Reform.

World Health Organization (WHO). (2006). *Maternal health*. Retrieved from http://www.who.int/topics/maternal_health/en/

CHAPTER 5

# Women, Aging, and Residential Long-Term Care

MORGAN SEELEY

Over 30 years have passed since Daniel Jay Baum (1977) used the term "warehouses for death" to describe the state of residential long-term care in Canada. Concerned about the rising numbers of older people being placed in long-term care institutions, Baum, like many scholars, activists, and social critics, associated residential care with social exclusion and age- and ability-based discrimination. His work made visible the poor quality of care provided in long-term care institutions and the "fragmented, underfinanced, and underutilized" state of home and community-based care services (1977, 9). Today, long-term care (LTC) has re-emerged as a "hot topic" in the popular media. This time, it is constructed as a public health care "crisis" caused by the "boomer tsunami," inciting fears that we will have neither the financial nor the human resources to sustain state-supported residential long-term care services. Although the validity of this line of reasoning is questionable (see Armstrong et al., 2009a; Armstrong, 2010), it has put residential LTC on the agenda of many policy-makers and researchers in Canada.

The purpose of this chapter is to encourage researchers and

policy-makers to attend to women, gender, and diversity when it comes to issues of residential LTC, not only because women are overrepresented as residents, paid care workers, and unpaid care providers in long-term care, but because issues central to discussions of residential LTC have differing impacts on women and are experienced differently by particular groups of men and women. In order to demonstrate the importance and usefulness of approaching residential LTC with women, gender, and diversity in mind, we draw largely on Canadian research and policy that considers residential LTC an issue for women. We look specifically at services provided outside of hospital and aimed at older people in order to reflect the current focus in policy and the popular media. We also draw on insights gathered over the course of a three-day workshop organized in 2007 by Women and Health Care Reform called "Designing Long-Term Facility Care for Women" and *A Place to Call Home: Long-Term Care in Canada* (Armstrong et al., 2009b), the book developed out of the panel presentations given at this workshop.

Recognizing the paucity of information on residential LTC, we begin to fill the gap by discussing why it should be understood as a women's issue. We examine the impact of long-term care reforms on women, attending to both similarities and differences among groups of women as residents, paid and unpaid workers, and as family members and friends. We end by considering the future of residential LTC research and policy in Canada.

## An Overview of Residential LTC in Canada

While a full description of residential LTC services in Canada is beyond the scope of this chapter (for more information, see Alexander, 2002; Banerjee, 2009; Berta et al., 2006), we use the term to describe a wide range of health and social services, policies, and programs that serve those who require ongoing care for indefinite lengths of time (Banerjee, 2009). Residential long-term care (also called "institutional" care) is defined in contrast to long-term care services that take place in homes and communities, although some services cross these boundaries. Currently, research and policy documents tend to use this term to describe services aimed at the aging population even though some institutions provide long-term care for populations under 65. For example, some non-senior adults and children with psychiatric, cognitive, emotional, or physical disabilities live in various forms of residential care. Residential LTC also tends to be distinguished from other forms of senior housing such as retirement homes or apartments for seniors because they are constructed with the explicit purpose of providing health care services such as access to 24-hour nursing care. However, this distinction becomes murky as health care services are increasingly provided in living arrangements for the aging that are not provincially or territorially funded, approved, or licensed.

Residential LTC in Canada differs across the country, owing in large part to diverse provincial and territorial histories (Alexander, 2002; Banerjee, 2009). What services are available, what they are called, what levels of care are provided, who provides what services, who pays and how much varies greatly between and within provincial and territorial jurisdictions. This diversity may be related to the precarious position long-term care holds as a public system. Unlike many primary health care services, long-term care is an extended health care service not explicitly covered under the *Canada Health Act*. Residential LTC is not fully insured by any province or territory in Canada, although at present, all provinces and territories contribute some funding to long-term care (Canadian Healthcare Association [CHA], 2009).

The direction of long-term care reforms in Canada both mimic and are affected by larger social and health care reforms, which since the 1970s have been characterized by neo-liberal discourses and practices. Recent provincial and territorial long-term care reforms, while differing according to location, are largely about containing the public costs of long-term care. Such reforms—supported

by notions of improved efficiencies and service coordination, economic and social accountability, and greater consumer choice—
have taken multiple forms. But what they have in common is they
are all versions of privatization. Similar to the five forms of health
care privatization Pat Armstrong discusses in the Introduction,
LTC reforms—such as the closure of psychiatric and chronic-care
hospitals, policies aimed at keeping people at home until the costs
of home support outweigh the costs of residential care; the closure
of publicly owned long-term care facilities; the replacement of
residential care beds with supportive housing and assisted living
arrangements; the contracting out of food, cleaning, laundry, and
other services provided within residential LTC settings to private
companies; and the expansion of private for-profit homes—have
effectively privatized the organization and delivery of services,
the work involved in LTC, and the costs of and the responsibility
for residential LTC.

## Challenges to Research and Policy on Gender, Aging, and Residential LTC

The prominence of a particular set of beliefs about the aging population may explain the lack of public outcry over the current state
of residential LTC, which is described by Leach and colleagues as
"a sector ignored as it suffers some of the worst impacts of health
care underfunding and restructuring" (2006, 1). Armstrong (2010)
argues that false assumptions about the aging population are used
to justify efforts to privatize long-term care services. Armstrong
suggests that by perpetuating myths that the aging population is
more dependent than other age groups, that seniors do not contribute to society, and that future cohorts of the aging population
will require levels of health care that we cannot afford, we are
reinforcing discrimination against older people instead of coming
up with ways to ensure they are treated with dignity and respect.
    Feminist social gerontologists (see Calasanti & Slevin, 2006)

remind us that discourses of old age are not gender-neutral. Ideals of feminine beauty largely devalue old women and their bodies, but beliefs about women's caregiving roles mean that aging women, despite being constructed as weak, sick, and dependent, are often conscripted into unpaid care work (King, 2006).

Grenier and Hanley (2007) discuss the ways in which gendered notions of frailty, specifically the discriminatory construction of older women as small, fragile, and powerless, are reinforced and materialized via health and social care services. Not only do these messages devalue older women and construct their bodies as "failing," but they are used to ration access to services, which are based on narrowly constructed notions of biomedical and functional need. Older women who resist or fail to comply with these stereotypes may risk losing access to formal LTC services (Grenier & Hanley, 2007).

While negative constructions of older people, particularly women, may act as a barrier to the development of residential LTC that emphasizes dignity and respect, it is also clear that within many health research communities, issues of residential LTC are not on the main agenda. Even feminist health researchers have been slow to examine the issue. Instead, long-term care policy and research is largely focused on home and community care. This disparity may be accounted for by several factors. First, since the 1980s, "aging in place" strategies, propped up by notions of self-determination, community participation, citizenship, and fiscal responsibility, have effectively moved care from institutions to households, where it is most often done by women and paid for by individuals and their family members. Accordingly, women's health researchers tend to focus their efforts on examining and critiquing the worsening working conditions, economic and health disparities experienced by women home care workers, as well as the financial, social, and health-related costs to women of a system that increasingly relies on unpaid gendered care provision (Neysmith, 1997; Neysmith & Aronson, 1997; Denton, Zeytinoglu, Webb & Lian, 1999).

Second, disability rights advocates and scholars have encouraged an emphasis on community and home-based long-term care programs and services, given a view of deinstitutionalization and independent living as necessary to the full social inclusion of people with disabilities. But the closure of psychiatric and chronic-care hospitals in particular was not and continues not to be complemented by the development of adequate publicly funded community-based supports and services. This has led in some cases to trans-institutionalization (the movement of people with disabilities into other forms of institutional facilities, including correctional facilities, hospital wards, and long-term care homes) and/or in many cases the downloading of care to private homes, communities, and to the streets. The focus on independent living may contribute to residential care being viewed as a last and least desirable option. It may also mean that those who continue to live in residential facilities fall through the gaps in critical disability policy and research.

Armstrong and Banerjee (2009) argue that the invisibility of residential LTC in research and policy is also related to its construction in terms of failure—the failure of medicine to cure disability and illness, the failure of families to provide care, and the failure of individuals to care for themselves. Drawing on Armstrong and Armstrong's (2008) discussion of how the movement of care from institutions to the home constitutes several forms of privatization, it becomes clear that constructing residential LTC in this way may actually threaten the health and well-being of women. They argue that a shift in where care is provided assumes that all people have homes and that homes are safe places for women who both require and provide care. But it also rests on gendered assumptions that as natural care providers, women have always cared in the home despite evidence that the kinds of care now required of women (e.g., using catheters and oxygen masks) was traditionally done elsewhere. Shifting care to the home rests on assumptions that those who require care want to live alone or with family members, and that families and women in particular want to provide care and have the resources to do so.

An explanation for the lack of research and policy that examines women and gender in residential LTC may relate to the construction of long-term care as a discrete set of medical services, tasks, or interventions. Penning and Votova (2009) are particularly weary of biomedically oriented approaches to health and aging, arguing that a cure-oriented Canadian health care system cannot address the needs of an aging population. Instead, as Armstrong and Banerjee (2009) have argued, residential long-term care is more appropriately approached from perspectives that emphasize social care and view care as a set of relationships: "It would be a model that incorporates medicine, but that also promotes dignity and respect by recognizing the context of individuals' lives, the contributions and skills of providers, and the importance of social relations as well as social meanings" (p. 24).

Finally, it may be that while research on residential LTC has blossomed in response to notions of the boomer tsunami, the dominance of medical approaches to this issue—a perspective that has historically ignored issues of gender, sex, and diversity—means that it has not been well identified as a women's issue. According to Johnson, Greaves, and Repta (2009), clinical and biomedical approaches to health research and policy have generally not attended to sex and gender or have erroneously conflated these terms. When it comes to more individually oriented studies on residential LTC, such as those emphasizing biomedicine and health promotion, sex- and gender-related similarities and differences are not often recorded or reported, even in cases where these data are readily available.

There are exceptions and these exceptions support notions that even when residential LTC is not approached with a focus on social relations, sex and gender differences emerge. For example, female LTC residents report more back pain than their male counterparts (D'Astolfo & Humphreys, 2006), and studies examining nutrient intake among LTC residents suggest that men and women have different kinds of deficiencies (Lengyel, Whiting & Zello, 2008; Lengyel, Zello, Smith & Whiting, 2003; Fratesi et al.,

2009). Sex and gender may also play a role in the success of health promotion programs run by LTC homes. For example, health promotion strategies aimed at increasing the physical activity levels of LTC residents (a population that reports particularly low levels of vigorous activity) may be enhanced by understanding barriers related to gender roles. Weeks et al. (2008) explain that older women who use LTC services associate low participation in physical activity to historic patterns of inactivity. It is argued that women's dual roles as paid workers and family care providers in their earlier years make regular exercise difficult and this acts as a barrier to participation later in life.

These examples from health promotion and biomedical research support the need for research that fully addresses differences among those impacted by residential LTC. As has been argued by Johnson, Greaves, and Repta (2009), approaching health research with a gender and diversity lens can improve the quality of research by making the evidence more comprehensive. It may support economic and quality-of-life concerns by ensuring services and programs are appropriate to the needs of multiple groups of seniors, as well as to their paid and unpaid care providers. And it may contribute to social justice by identifying disparities in access to and experiences of residential LTC.

# Residential LTC as a Women's Issue

The impact of LTC reforms and the messages that support them are not felt evenly across the population. Statistics suggest that only 7 percent of the population over 65 years of age live in residential care facilities (Statistics Canada, 2007), but the effects are felt on the many more who support a family member or friend and/or provide paid or unpaid care in these settings. Residential LTC is of fundamental concern to women, given that they comprise over 63 percent of residents living in all residential care facilities and over 70 percent of those living in homes for the aged (Statistics Canada,

2010). Women's higher life expectancy, higher risk of dementia, and greater likelihood of living alone in old age are often used to explain their overrepresentation in residential LTC. However, gender-based inequities—such as higher rates of disability and poverty, lower average socio-economic status, and poorer access to informal community-based care (Penning & Votova, 2009)— mean women are more likely to rely on such services.

There are significant differences within groups of women who use residential LTC services. According to Statistics Canada (2010) data, almost 50 percent of women living in residential care facilities are the "oldest old," meaning they are 85 years of age or older. Admission requirements also mean that residents are likely to have complex health issues, severe impairments, or are technology dependent (Armstrong et al., 2009a; CHA, 2009). Residents are more likely to be unmarried, widowed, separated, or divorced (Asakawa et al., 2009); and the likelihood of transitioning from independent living arrangements to residential care increases when women lack publicly provided home care. A lack of informal home and community supports and lower levels of wealth also make residing in LTC a greater possibility (Sarma et al. 2009). Research also indicates that racialized and immigrant women are less likely to use residential LTC, leading to questions about equitable access to services, as well as the cultural appropriateness of existing services (Asakawa et al., 2009; Koehn, 2009).

LTC services are also an issue for women because we provide the overwhelming majority of paid and unpaid long-term care (Armstrong & Banerjee, 2009). Studies carried out in various provinces suggest that over 90 percent of staff working in residential care facilities are women—a significant number of whom are from racialized and/or migrant communities (Armstrong et al., 2009a; Cohen, 2009). Furthermore, women provide a significant amount of unpaid care as family members and friends of residents, as formal volunteers supplementing the work of paid providers, and as workers, many of whom do unpaid overtime and work through breaks to help fill gaps in care.

# Women and the Privatization of Residential LTC

As a whole, women's health advocates and others view the current direction of LTC reform as bad for the health of women. Characterized by privatization (the privatization of the organization and delivery of services, the privatization of residential LTC work, the privatization of costs for care, and the privatization of responsibility for care), these reforms impact women's access to residential LTC services, the quality of care they receive as residents, the quality of women's work environments, and the ability of women to support family and friends who require this form of care. The growth of privatization occurs in the context of an overall reduction in state involvement in funding and provision of long-term health and social care, and an absence of policies and programs that ensure equitable access to high-quality residential LTC. The closure of publicly owned facilities, reductions in the number of publicly funded LTC beds, the contracting out of services to for-profit firms, and policies aimed at downloading the costs for care to individuals, families, and communities further perpetuate the privatization of these services.

**WOMEN'S ACCESS TO RESIDENTIAL LTC: THE ROLE OF THE STATE**
The privatization of residential LTC is supported by the precarious position LTC services hold under the *Canada Health Act*, where it is considered an "extended health care service," meaning that only some aspects of care are fully insured. The portions of LTC services that are privatized become the responsibility of residents and/or their family members. Privatizing the costs of care is a particular issue for older women in Canada, especially if they are single, divorced, or otherwise unattached; senior women report significantly lower average income than their male counterparts (Statistics Canada, 2009, Table 1-1).

The personal costs associated with residential LTC are also an issue for older women because of gender differences in sources of income. According to Denton and Boos (2007), many women have difficulty building assets such as pensions because the role they play in unpaid caregiving limits their involvement in the paid labour force. Not surprisingly, women over the age of 65 are more likely than men to rely on government subsidies such as Old Age Security Pensions and the Guaranteed Income Supplement (CHA, 2009). The scant personal allowance remaining after monthly facility fees are paid to residential LTC facilities means that residents relying on government funding are unable to cover essential expenses not covered by facility fees such as hearing aids, dentures, specialized wheelchairs, and personal hygiene products (Canadian Union of Public Employees [CUPE], 2009). The issue of cost is compounded for more recent immigrant seniors, who are less likely to be eligible for full subsidies.

Since the provinces and territories are largely responsible for deciding which aspects of long-term care are publicly funded, the private costs of care differ greatly (and inequitably) across jurisdictions. A recent examination of the personal costs of residential LTC across the provinces of Canada indicated large disparities not only geographically but in combination with income level, marital status, and, in Quebec, assets holdings (Fernandes & Spencer, 2010). For example, among unmarried residents,

> Those with very low incomes pay about one quarter more for their care if they live in Newfoundland or Prince Edward Island rather than Nova Scotia, those with low incomes pay half again as much if they live in Ontario rather than British Columbia and two-thirds more if they live in Newfoundland or Prince Edward Island, while those with average incomes or higher pay approximately twice as much in five provinces (British Columbia, Manitoba, Nova Scotia, New Brunswick, and Prince Edward Island) as in Quebec, and close to three times as much in Newfoundland. (pp. 310–311)

Such disparities lead some advocates to suggest that in contrast to the principles of the *Canada Health Act*, both personal wealth and geographic location greatly affect access to residential LTC. But what is not often discussed is the gendered impact of these disparities. Since older women tend to have less income and are more likely to live alone, jurisdictional disparities in personal costs may mean that older women residing in LTC are unable to move closer to family members and friends (Fernandes & Spencer, 2010), while others in need of residential care may feel pressure to leave their family and community in order to get affordable care.

The situation is particularly dire for Aboriginal peoples over 65, 54 percent of whom are women (Statistics Canada, 2007). Eshkakogan and Ernest Khalema (2009) remind us that Aboriginal peoples' poorer access to health-promoting conditions such as housing, employment, and health services mean they are at greater risk of requiring LTC services. Many of the factors associated with entrance into residential forms of care—such as chronic illness and disability, low income, a paucity of publicly funded, community-based LTC services, and poor housing—are experienced at higher rates among Aboriginal peoples. Yet they face significant barriers in terms of access to care, including a lack of LTC facilities located in First Nations communities, particularly of facilities that provide high levels of health and personal care (Assembly of First Nations [AFN], 2005). Conflicts over who is responsible for funding and providing various LTC services for on- and off-reserve, status and non-status Aboriginal peoples (AFN, 2005; Eshkakogan & Ernest Khalema, 2009), a lack of coordination of available services, and a lack of services that provide culturally competent care (e.g., those that integrate Aboriginal practices and understandings of health, healing, and dying) (Eshkakogan & Ernest Khalema, 2009) all suggest that when it comes to long-term care, this population is falling through the cracks.

The retrenchment of the state from residential LTC provision also perpetuates the privatization of care. A clear example is the overwhelming number of policies aimed at shifting long-term care from institutions to communities and homes. Often justified as strategies that give seniors the option and opportunity to "age in place" (Shapiro & Seeley, 2009), in the absence of adequate home care and community supports, Aronson and Neysmith (1997) and others (see Armstrong, 2007; Shapiro & Seeley, 2009; Williams & Crooks, 2008) have long viewed "deinstitutionalization" strategies such as the closure of chronic-care facilities and hospitals and reductions to the number of publicly operated nursing home beds as instances of privatizing the costs of, responsibility for, and work involved in long-term care. These policies clearly have an impact on women, for whom the movement from institution to community and home-based care has often meant conscription into the provision of medically and technologically complex care (see Chapter 6 for more on care at home).

Privatization strategies also affect those who continue to require residential forms of long-term care. One example is the push to develop assisted living facilities. Shapiro and Seeley (2009) use the example of Alberta, where the province has encouraged the development of supportive housing units under the guise of providing seniors with more choices when it comes to care. To do this, "services previously provided by nursing homes were being 'unbundled' by separating the costs of health from housing and support services, and limiting the number of nursing home beds" (p. 61).

Unbundling services allows various seniors' living arrangements to provide a number of care services that residents can "choose" from, depending on their individual needs. But the unbundling of services and the expansion of assisted living and supportive housing facilities may not be in the best interests of women. A report by the National Union of Public and General Employees (NUPGE, 2007) argues that while the original model of assisted living aimed to provide home-like atmospheres that gave residents greater control while offering support with social and health care, "The original vision has been largely co-opted by commercial operators looking for a high return on investments" (p. 17). The push to assisted living is an instance of downloading the costs of care to residents and their families. While some services may be covered publicly by home care, others must be paid for by individuals, often at high prices (NUPGE, 2007). These arrangements may be largely unaffordable and therefore inaccessible to many older women. And Shapiro and Seeley (2009) raise concerns about the quality of care provided in these spaces, given the provinces and territories' lack of commitment to approving, licensing, and monitoring assisted living and supportive housing.

The impact on women as paid care workers is also a central concern. Without regulation, owners are not required to provide staff with particular levels of training and supervision, and staff may be required to provide levels of care they are not properly trained to provide (Shapiro & Seeley, 2009). The report by NUPGE (2007) also reminds us that in diverting funds from residential LTC facilities to supportive and assisted living arrangements, provinces like Alberta have witnessed cuts in staffing levels in residential LTC facilities. This leaves direct care staff overburdened and the quality of care compromised.

Of similar concern is the expansion of private, for-profit ownership of residential LTC facilities, often referred to as long-term care homes. While the extent of this growth varies greatly across the country with, for example, Manitoba reporting 28 percent of all approved beds in homes for the aged as private, for-profit compared with almost 61 percent in Ontario (Statistics Canada, 2010, tables 1-7, 1-8), we are clearly witnessing large increases in corporate investment in residential long-term care. For example, in 1988, 48.7 percent of LTC facilities in Canada had private, for-profit ownership (Penning & Votova, 2009). This number increased to 54.5 percent in 2007–2008 (Statistics Canada, 2010, Table 1-1). Recent Statistics Canada data (2010, Table 1-1) indicate that while 44 percent of all approved beds in homes for the aged in Canada are for-profit, only 0.2 percent are operated by municipal, provincial, or territorial governments (currently, the federal government does not operate any homes for the aged).

## WOMEN AND THE RISE OF FOR-PROFIT RESIDENTIAL LTC

Women's health scholars and advocates are particularly concerned about the impact of a rise of for-profit homes on the quality of care provided to residents and the conditions of work for paid providers. Pitters (2002) argues that a lack of sophisticated studies on this issue and the difficulty of defining quality make claims of better quality difficult to argue. But McGrail and colleagues (2007) suggest that publicly operated facilities provide better health outcomes for residents, citing research using hospital admission data from Manitoba and British Columbia that show higher overall hospital admission rates (Shapiro & Tate, 2005) and higher admission rates for dehydration, pneumonia, and anemia (McGregor et al., 2006) among residents living in for-profit residential LTC. These higher hospital admission rates for for-profit residences may be explained by disparities in staffing levels between government-operated and for-profit facilities, where in order to make a profit, budgets for staffing are kept at a minimum (McGrail et al., 2007).

Indeed, several North American studies indicate that for-profit LTC facilities generally have lower staffing levels than not-for-profit facilities, particularly when it comes to direct care provision (CUPE, 2009). This is an issue for women as residents because, as a report by CHA (2009) argues, staffing levels are the "key to quality." A summary of studies examining the relationship between the amount of direct care provided to residents and a range of physical and emotional health indicators suggests that lower staffing levels are associated with adverse outcomes such as incontinence, falls, weight loss, dehydration, fractures, pressure ulcers, and aggressive behaviours (see CUPE, 2009). Low staffing levels may correspond with excessive workloads for staff, which means no time to care for residents—no time for essential tasks such as toileting, ensuring residents get a comfortable bath and have clean clothes and linens, no time to maintain a clean living (and working) environment, and no time for social care such as providing emotional support, talking or walking with residents (Armstrong et al., 2009a).

Lower staffing levels can negatively impact the work environment of paid care workers in long-term care, the overwhelming majority of whom are women. Cohen's (2009) discussion of research on this topic conducted in British Columbia indicates a relationship between staffing levels and the health and safety of workers in residential long-term care. Specifically, higher staffing levels for direct care staff translate to lower injury rates among providers. Armstrong and colleagues' (2009a) examination of working conditions in residential long-term care in Canada and Scandinavia indicates that workers in Canada identify the need for more staff as an issue above all other concerns. In this study, inadequate staffing is associated with excessive workloads that compromised the ability of workers to provide residents with dignified, compassionate care. Not surprisingly, LTC workers in Canada often reported feeling inadequate and regularly experienced mental fatigue, loss of sleep, and physical exhaustion (Armstrong et al., 2009a).

There is also some indication that LTC workers in for-profit facilities receive lower wages than those employed in government-operated facilities. Licensed practical nurses (LPNs) working in for-profit homes report lower incomes than those in non-profit homes (Armstrong et al., 2009a), and despite difficulties in accessing data on this topic, there is reason to believe this is also the case for personal support workers (PSWs) (Armstrong et al., 2009a). Lower wages not only reinforce women's poorer access to the conditions necessary for health and well-being, but they may cost the system more. A study examining sickness absenteeism among health care workers in British Columbia (Gorman, Yu & Alamgir, 2010) found that those with lower hourly wages were more likely to take sickness absences.

The effects of low wages are not gender-neutral. Describing low wages among residential LTC workers, we are reminded that "Clearly these wage differences are not about the nature of the job. The low wage rates reflect the search for profit. They also reflect, especially for PSWs, the attitude toward the work and the women who do this work" (Armstrong et al., 2009a, 87). Indeed, assumptions about care work being "women's work" may be used to maintain low salaries, high workloads, and unhealthy working conditions within residential LTC homes.

This is not to say that the care and work environments of facilities owned by public and private not-for-profit sectors ensure the health and well-being of women. The implementation of practices widely used by for-profit sectors to deliver and organize care makes it exceedingly difficult for *all* facilities to provide good-quality living and working conditions. Such reforms reflect assumptions that the private sector has developed methods of organizing and delivering care that are more efficient and effective. Some examples of the privatization of the organization and delivery of services in residential LTC include the downloading of work from higher paid to lesser paid providers; the contracting out of services in public LTC facilities to for-profit companies; and the division of care provided in LTC facilities into discrete, measurable, and standardized tasks.

### PRIVATIZING THE RESIDENTIAL LTC WORKPLACE: THE IMPACTS ON WOMEN

Hallgrimsdottir, Teghtsoonian, and Brown (2008) emphasize the gendered impact of downloading care work to less skilled and more poorly paid care workers. They argue that efforts to reduce the costs of health care are linked to a "gendered occupational hierarchy," which rests on assumptions that the social aspects of care are unskilled and "natural" for women. The assumption that care work can be done by those with less training justifies the lower wages of personal support workers (PSWs), who provide the majority of direct care work in residential LTC. Despite increasing workloads and an increase in the complexity of tasks required of PSWs, they continue to be paid less than registered nurses, receive most of their training on the job, and are not well regulated (Armstrong et al., 2009a). Armstrong and colleagues (2009a) remind us that the undervaluation of care work in residential LTC has a racist component that interacts with these gendered assumptions. They provide the example of immigrant women who, despite having their credentials from abroad unrecognized, are considered able to work in long-term care in Canada. Similarly, in their examination of immigrant nurses employed in home and residential long-term care, Bourgeault and Wrede (2008) confirm that

> the migration process is linked to the devaluing of care (in terms of wages and working conditions), which is in turn connected to recent neo-liberal reforms, pushing some nurses from the country in which they were trained to better remuneration and working conditions somewhere else. (p. S22)

The contracting out of services provided in both for-profit and not-for-profit LTC facilities is a second example of the privatization of work in residential LTC that has particular impacts on women as providers and residents. Stinson's (2006) discussion of contracting out hospital and residential LTC workers who provide cleaning, food, and laundry services in British Columbia suggests that this form of privatization is not good for the health and well-being of care workers. Contracting out is associated with cuts in wages and benefits, less predictable work schedules, and exhaustive workloads that lead to personal health issues. A CUPE (2009) report also links contracting out to "inadequate training, job insecurity, and high turnover" (p. 57). However, very little research has focused specifically on the conditions of work for women who provide care that is often categorized as "ancillary" to health care work. This is particularly the case for residential LTC, where studies have overwhelmingly focused on nurses and, to a lesser extent, personal support workers. Our own experiences doing research in residential long-term care provide anecdotal indications that ancillary workers may attempt to fill some of the gaps left in the provision of social care by making time to chat with residents and providing some emotional support.

The adoption of for-profit management strategies and practices in residential LTC is also an issue for women. Armstrong and colleagues (2009a) use the term "assembly line care" to describe caring labour in LTC homes that "becomes a task-oriented function to be done in the shortest time possible" (p. 109). But speeding up care may not be in the best interests of women. A report by NUPGE (2007) summarizes several of the concerns associated with how residential long-term care is delivered in the current context, providing examples like residents having to wait for intimate care, too few baths, inadequate fluid intake, failure to provide appropriate rehabilitation services, lack of exercise and counselling services, decrepit living facilities, and heavy workloads for staff. These all translate into a lack of time to provide good-quality care.

The movement to this form of delivery and organization ultimately leads to "the rationing of social-emotional care" (CUPE, 2009, 37). Because evidence indicates that under this model workers are unable to meet standardized times to complete discrete care tasks (see Armstrong and Daly, 2004), the social and emotional aspects of care are rationed (CUPE, 2009). A survey of direct care providers in Ontario, Nova Scotia, and Manitoba (Armstrong et al., 2009a) report that social care is often left undone: " A third [of workers] say they often do not have time to chat to patients or to take them out of their confined physical spaces. Less than a quarter say the essential emotional support required by these residents is never left undone, and the same is the case for chatting" (pp. 105–106). Paid workers also report doing unpaid labour such as working through breaks and taking on additional shifts to cope with inadequate staffing levels, only some of which they report being compensated for (see Armstrong et al., 2009a, 69).

It may not be surprising that under these conditions, paid workers in residential long-term care report particularly high rates of injury and sickness. A study of health care workers in three health regions in British Columbia revealed that "CAs [care aides] in the LTC sector were found to be at three times higher risk for all injury and MSIs [musculoskeletal injury] compared to RNs in acute care" (Alamgir, Yu, Chavoshi & Ngan, 2008, 350). While an analysis of gender is not presented in this study, it is important to note that of the 3,000 CAs surveyed, over 90 percent were women.

Armstrong and Daly (2004) and Armstrong and colleagues (2009a) have also demonstrated that under current practices, workers in residential long-term care experience various forms of violence, including physical, verbal, sexual, and racialized violence. Personal support workers report higher levels of violence from residents and their family members than other direct care workers, but almost all direct care workers surveyed (RNs, LPNs, and PSWs) report experiencing physical violence in their workplace. Even dietary staff and housekeeping staff report violence, albeit in much lower numbers (Armstrong et al., 2009a).

## WOMEN AND THE PROVISION OF UNPAID RESIDENTIAL LTC

The privatization of residential care, including the adoption of for-profit managerial practices, the contracting out of services, and downloading of care work to lesser paid care workers, clearly impacts both the quality of care provided to residents and the quality of the paid work environment experienced by paid care workers. But it also has an impact on women who are family members and friends of LTC residents. Heavier workloads for paid staff, not enough time to provide social care, and more frequent absenteeism from sickness may mean that family members have to fill the gaps in care. As a report by CUPE (2009) puts it, "the general pattern of underfunding, deregulation and privatization of residential long-term care in Canada means that already-burdened families are being asked to take on more responsibility for their loved-one's care" (p. 30). However, we know little about those who provide unpaid care to family and friends in residential LTC, especially in comparison to the wealth of research on women as informal care providers in the home. What we do know is that women are more likely than men to provide unpaid care to family and friends living in facilities. And we also know that

126

families play an essential role in the quality of life experienced by LTC residents.

Henderson's (2002) list of care work provided by family and friends provides some indication of the extent to which unpaid care is relied upon to ensure the well-being of residents. Family and friends are responsible for purchasing clothing, supplies, and other needs not provided by facilities; assisting with meals and providing personal care while visiting with residents; providing emotional support and comfort; managing health care provision outside the facility, such as accompanying residents to family doctors and specialist appointments; and acting as an advocate for residents. Research conducted by the Ontario Health Coalition (OHC, 2008) also noted the assistance provided to non-filial residents who do not have family members and friends to fill gaps in care.

There are indications that the structure of the care environment directly impacts family members' engagement with paid workers. Gladstone, Dupuis, and Wexler's (2007) longitudinal study of family members of residents in Ontario demonstrated that high staff workloads and staff turnover negatively impact relationships with family members.

Family members are not the only unpaid care providers who fill the gap in care. While research on the contributions of this group is extremely scant, it is clear that formal volunteers play an increasingly important role in the provision of social care to LTC residents. Even less understood is the extent to which residents in long-term care provide unpaid care to one another. These are clearly areas that require further exploration.

# Women, Gender, and the Future of Residential LTC

We have reflected on recent LTC reforms, arguing that movements to privatize the costs, delivery, organization, and work involved in residential LTC may undermine the health and well-being of women as residents, paid and unpaid workers, and family and friends. In this final section, we suggest the need for more gender- and diversity-focused research and policy analyses.

It is clear that residential LTC is becoming a "hot topic" as panic over an aging baby boomer population spreads. We feel some hesitation in emphasizing demographic trends in residential LTC as they tend to be used in the current political and economic environment to rationalize public cutbacks to the provision of residential LTC services and the movement toward privatization of care more generally. For example, demographic changes indicating that the upcoming generation of senior women will have more income, better health, and higher education may be used to benefit senior women by undermining stereotypes about them as frail, dependent, and even a burden to the public health care system. Yet the same assumptions about this generation of older women is also used to divert funding to community-based models of residential care, which may be harmful to women with high or complex care needs, those who lack informal supports, and/or who cannot afford the costs of care.

And while older women (particularly the oldest old) are likely to continue to comprise the majority of LTC residents, it is also important to remember that they are not the only seniors who use residential LTC services. Reports of a closing gender gap in life expectancy may influence the development of policy and research on men and residential LTC. This area may be well warranted as current policies and programs reflecting the interests and concerns of men in residential LTC are rare (CHA, 2009). There is evidence that male residents have different health concerns and risks than their female counterparts. For example, Voyer and colleagues (2007) have reported a greater prevalence of minor injuries resulting from falls among senior male residents. The provision of stereotypically female activities in residential LTC also comes up in the literature and is an issue that, if changed, could benefit the quality of activities for both male and female residents.

Younger adults between the ages of 18 and 65 also comprise a small number of those living in residential long-term care. While we know little about this group, criteria for entrance into residential LTC means this group is likely to have particularly high medical and other care needs, and unlikely to have family and other unpaid care providers to fill the gaps in care. One study of non-senior adults with traumatic brain injuries living in long-term care for seniors in Ontario (Colantonio, Howse & Patel, 2010) reported that this group requires a great deal of assistance with activities of daily living, a large percentage are classified as having "challenging behaviours," and approximately 12 percent have substance abuse issues. Others have suggested that "positive outcomes [for non-senior residents] are not usually realized due to feelings of isolation and boredom" (Pitters, 2002, 179). And anecdotal evidence suggests the need for different social and recreational programs to meet the interests and needs of younger residents.

The rapid ethnic diversification of seniors in some areas of Canada also raises questions about equitable access and the availability of culturally appropriate residential LTC services. Koehn (2009) examined access to continuing care services among immigrant and ethnic minority seniors who associated themselves with the Hispanic, Vietnamese, and Punjabi seniors' communities in Vancouver. These older people reported barriers to LTC services, such as difficult family dynamics, that had resulted from the process of migration—specifically their dependence on children for financial support. Concerns over the availability of food consistent with their culture and religion, access to religious services, and language barriers when seniors undergo assessments for access by health care workers are also a concern. This may be a particular issue for older women immigrants who, Koehn suggests, are less likely than men to be literate in their own language in addition to English. A fear of loneliness and discomfort living in residential LTC facilities where the majority of residents are White and English-speaking are also reported barriers.

Research in the area of ethnic seniors is scarce, but the indication that immigrant and ethnic minority seniors experience barriers to LTC suggests the need for culturally appropriate LTC services that actively promote anti-racism. Part of the issue may be the assumption on the part of service providers and the mainstream public that immigrant and ethnic minority seniors will be taken care of by their own communities (Koehn, 2009). Residential LTC providers may have a lot to learn from ethnoculturally specific community organizations that have long established culturally appropriate LTC services (CHA, 2009), but such initiatives should not remain the sole responsibility of these groups.

Concerns about the provision of residential LTC to lesbian, gay, bisexual, transgender, and transsexual (LGBTT) older people have also emerged in popular media and among advocacy groups. There is little Canadian research that explicitly examines issues regarding access to health and social services among LGBTT seniors in general. But research outside of Canada reports that gay and lesbian seniors are more likely to delay entrance into residential long-term care (Addis et al., 2009). Viewing institutionalization as threatening to LGBTT older people is warranted, given that gay and lesbian seniors may experience being "outed," neglected, threatened, and even physically and/or sexually assaulted (Addis et al., 2009).

Moore (2009) suggests that transsexual individuals he has worked with are particularly fearful of residential LTC. They worry about being seen as "freaks" by workers performing intimate care, having to go back into the closet, and not having their needs met. Efforts like those of the Homes for the Aged Division of the City of Toronto to develop objectives and protocols for providing safe and positive residential LTC environments for queer residents are important first steps (see Moore, 2009).

The changing demographics of paid workers in residential LTC also warrant further consideration. One area of concern is the age of residential LTC workers. According to Armstrong and Daly

(2004), the current generation of female workers, particularly RNs, are middle-aged and older:

> Many stay because they remember the days when care was there and hope to see those days return. The rewards come from their commitment to care and their extra work to make up for the care deficit. When this generation retires, the next may be unwilling to take on work that seems to provide few rewards in terms of pay, security or resident satisfaction. (p. 5)

Given the reports of violence, stress, injury, and unbearable workloads already discussed, the issue of poor worker retention is undeniable (see also Chapter 7, "Women's Work in Health Care").

The second area of interest is the ethnic diversification of LTC workers, specifically the increase in immigrant and/or racialized workers in particular regions in Canada. There are reasons to be concerned about the well-being of immigrant and/or racialized female care workers. Armstrong and colleagues (2009a) describe instances of racism experienced by residential LTC workers, particularly from residents. Bourgeault and colleagues (2010) also suggest that language barriers and differences in ethnic and cultural backgrounds can strain relationships between immigrant care workers and older recipients of residential and home-based LTC services. While many workers report positive relationships with care recipients, some relationships were characterized by discrimination on the basis of the carer's skin colour, accent, or language differences, most often expressed in the form of verbal abuse by older clients.

Finally, demographic trends among those who provide the majority of unpaid care to the aging population both as family members, or friends, and as formal volunteers will influence the future of residential LTC for seniors. Women's increasing participation in the paid workforce, the projected doubling of the ratio of older people to the number of working-age people over the next three to four decades (Organisation for Economic Co-operation and Development [OECD], 2005), and current trends in fertility rates and migration patterns (Doupe et al., 2006) all mean that many seniors will not be able to rely on unpaid supports to provide LTC. This also means that the reliance of residential LTC facilities on family and friends to fill gaps in care may be compromised.

It has also been argued that the social characteristics of future cohorts of seniors, many of whom act as formal volunteers in residential LTC, need to be better understood. Drawing on data from Volunteer Canada (2009), the CHA (2009) argues that while the number of seniors available to volunteer may increase as baby boomers age, this may not translate into more volunteers. Volunteer participation in residential LTC may be affected by the privatization of care organization and delivery. The direction of current reforms seems to reinforce aspects of volunteer work that are least preferred by upcoming cohorts of seniors, who complain about "unreasonable expectations, burnout, unreasonable deadlines, [and] absence of feedback and appreciation" (CHA, 2009, 101).

Changing demographics of future LTC residents, paid care workers, family, friends, and volunteers mean that residential LTC must also change. But the answer is not to "manufacture a crisis" over the future of public health care. Rather, we must work toward ensuring residential LTC is a good choice as opposed to a failure or the least desirable option. Given that residential LTC is a women's issue, one response is the development of research and policy that attends to gender and diversity. We hope we have demonstrated the potential of this lens to provide information central to the provision of residential LTC that is accessible and of high quality and promotes dignity and respect among and between residents, and paid and unpaid care providers.

# References

Addis, S., Davies, M., Greene, G., MacBride-Stewart, S. & Shepherd, M. (2009). The health, social care, and housing needs of lesbian, gay, bisexual, and transgender older people: A review of the literature. *Health and Social Care in the Community* 17(6), 647–658.

Alamgir, H., Yu, S., Chavoshi, N. & Ngan, K. (2008). Occupational injury among full-time, part-time, and casual health care workers. *Occupational Medicine* 58, 348–354.

Alexander, T. (2002). The history and evolution of long-term care in Canada. In M. Stephenson & E. Sawyer (Eds.), *Continuing the care: The issues and challenges for long-term care* (pp. 1–55). Ottawa: CHA Press.

Armstrong, P. (2007). Relocating care: Home care in Ontario. In M. Morrow, O. Hankivsky & C. Varcoe (Eds.), *Women's health in Canada: Critical perspectives on theory and policy* (pp. 528–553). Toronto: University of Toronto Press.

Armstrong, P. (2010, November). Manufactured crisis: The silver tsunami. Paper presented at the Ontario Health Coalition Manufactured crisis: The myth of medicare's unsustainability and what it means for Ontarians conference, Ontario Health Coalition, Toronto.

Armstrong, P. & Armstrong, H. (2008). *About Canada: Health care*. Winnipeg: Fernwood Publishing.

Armstrong, P. & Banerjee, A. (2009). Challenging questions: Designing long-term residential care with women in mind. In P. Armstrong et al. (Eds.), *A place to call home: Long-term care in Canada* (pp. 10–28). Winnipeg: Fernwood Publishing.

Armstrong, P., Banerjee, A., Szebehely, M., Armstrong, H., Daly, T. & Lafrance, S. (2009a). *They deserve better: The long-term care experience in Canada and Scandinavia*. Ottawa: CCPA.

Armstrong, P., Boscoe, M., Clow, B., Grant, K., Haworth-Brockman, M., Jackson, B., Pederson, A., Seeley, M. & Springer, J. (Eds.). (2009b). *A place to call home: Long-term care in Canada*. Winnipeg: Fernwood Publishing.

Armstrong, P. & Daly, T. (2004, July). *There are not enough hands: Conditions of Ontario's long-term care facilities*. Ottawa: CUPE. Retrieved from http://cupe.ca /updir/CUPELTC-ReportEng1.pdf

Aronson, J. & Neysmith, S.M. (1997). The retreat of the state and long-term care provision: Implications for frail elderly people, unpaid family carers, and paid home care workers. *Studies in Political Economy 53*, 37–66.

Asakawa, K., Feeny, D., Senthilselvan, A., Johnson, J.A. & Rolfson, D. (2009). Do the determinants of health differ between people living in the community and in institutions? *Social Science and Medicine 69*, 345–353.

Assembly of First Nations (AFN). (2005, June). *First Nations action plan on continuing care*. Retrieved from http://www.afn.ca/cmslib/general/CCAP.pdf

Banerjee, A. (2009). Long-term care in Canada: An overview. In P. Armstrong et al. (Eds.), *A place to call home: Long-term care in Canada* (pp. 28–57). Winnipeg: Fernwood Publishing.

Baum, D.J. (1977). *Warehouses for death: The nursing home industry*. Don Mills: Burns & MacEachern.

Berta, W., Laporte, A., Zarnett, D., Valdmanis, V. & Anderson, G. (2006). A pan-Canadian perspective on institutional long-term care. *Health Policy 79*, 175–194.

Bourgeault, I., Atanackovic, J., Rashid, A. & Parpia, R. (2010). Relations between immigrant care workers and older persons in home and long-term care. *Canadian Journal on Aging 29*(1), 109–118.

Bourgeault, I. & Wrede, S. (2008). Caring beyond borders: Comparing the relationship between work and migration patterns in Canada and Finland. *Canadian Journal of Public Health 99*(Suppl. 2), S22–S26.

Calasanti, T.M. & Slevin, K.F. (Eds.). (2006). *Age matters: Realigning feminist thinking*. New York: Routledge.

Canadian Healthcare Association (CHA). (2009). *New directions for facility-based long-term care*. Ottawa: CHA.

Canadian Union of Public Employees (CUPE). (2009). *Residential long-term care in Canada: Our vision for better seniors' care*. Ottawa: CUPE.

Cohen, M. (2009). What matters to women working in long-term care:

A union perspective. In P. Armstrong et al. (Eds.), *A place to call home: Long-term care in Canada* (pp. 97–103). Winnipeg: Fernwood Publishing.

Colantonio, A., Howse, D. & Patel, J. (2010). Young adults with traumatic brain injury in long-term care homes: A population-based study. *Brain Impairment 11*(1), 31–36.

D'Astolfo, C.J. & Humphreys, B.K. (2006). A record review of reported musculoskeletal pain in an Ontario long-term care facility. *BMC Geriatrics 6*(5). Retrieved from http://www.biomedcentral.com/content/pdf/1471-2318-6-5.pdf

Denton, M. & Boos, L. (2007). The gender wealth gap: Structural and material implications for later life. *Journal of Women and Aging 19*(3), 105–120.

Denton, M.A., Zeytinoglu, I.U., Webb, S. & Lian, J. (1999). Occupational health issues among employees of home care agencies. *Canadian Journal on Aging 18*(2), 154–181.

Doupe, M., Brownell, M., Kozyrskyj, A., Dik, N., Burchill, C., Dahl, M., Chateau, D., De Coster, C., Hinds, A. & Bodnarchuk, J. (2006, October). *Using administrative data to develop indicators of quality care in personal care homes.* Winnipeg: Manitoba Centre for Health Policy.

Eshkakogan, N. & Ernest Khalema, N. (2009). A contradictory image of need: Long-term facilitative care for First Nations. In P. Armstrong et al. (Eds.), *A place to call home: Long-term care in Canada* (pp. 66–78). Winnipeg: Fernwood Publishing.

Fernandes, N. & Spencer, B.G. (2010). The private costs of long-term care in Canada: Where you live matters. *Canadian Journal on Aging 29*(3), 307–316.

Fratesi, J.A., Hogg, R.C., Young-Newton, G.S., Patterson, A.C., Charkhzarin, P., Block Thomas, K., Sharratt, M.T. & Stark, K.D. (2009). Direct quantitation of omega-3 fatty acid intake of Canadian residents of a long-term care facility. *Applied Physiology, Nutrition, and Metabolism 34*, 1–9.

Gladstone, J.W., Dupuis, S.L. & Wexler, E. (2007). Ways that families engage with staff in long-term care facilities. *Canadian Journal on Aging 26*(4), 391–402.

Gorman, E., Yu, S. & Alamgir, H. (2010). When healthcare workers get sick: Exploring sickness absenteeism in British Columbia. *Work 35*, 117–123.

Grenier, A. & Hanley, J. (2007). Older women and "frailty": Aged, gendered, and embodied resistance. *Current Sociology 55*(2), 211–228.

Hallgrimsdottir, H.K., Teghtsoonian, K. & Brown, D. (2008). Public policy, caring practices, and gender in health care work. *Canadian Journal of Public Health 99*(Suppl. 2), S43–S47.

Henderson, K. (2002). Informal caregivers. In M. Stephenson & E. Sawyer (Eds.), *Continuing the care: The issues and challenges for long-term care* (pp. 267–290). Ottawa: CHA Press.

Johnson, J.L., Greaves, L. & Repta, R. (2009). Better science with sex and gender: Facilitating the use of a sex and gender-based analysis in health research. *International Journal for Equity in Health 8*(14). Retrieved from http://www.equityhealthj.com/content/8/1/14

King, N. (2006). The lengthening list of oppressions: Age relations and the feminist study of inequality. In T.M. Calasanti & K.F. Slevin (Eds.), *Age matters: Realigning feminist thinking* (pp. 47–74). New York: Routledge.

Koehn, S. (2009). Negotiating candidacy: Ethnic minority seniors' access to care. *Aging and Society 29*, 585–608.

Leach, B., Hallman, B., Joseph, G., Martin, N. & Marcotte, A. (2006). *The impact of patient classification systems on women front-line care workers in rural nursing homes*. Ottawa: Status of Women Canada.

Lengyel, C.O., Whiting, S.J. & Zello, G.A. (2008). Nutrient inadequacies among elderly residents of long-term care facilities. *Canadian Journal of Dietetic Practice and Research 69*(2), 82–88.

Lengyel, C.O., Zello, G.A., Smith, J.T. & Whiting, S.J. (2003). Evaluation of menu and food service practices of long-term care facilities of a health district in Canada. *Journal of Nutrition for the Elderly 22*(3), 29–42.

McGrail, K.M., McGregor, M.J., Cohen, M., Tate, R.B. & Ronald, L.A. (2007). For-profit versus not-for-profit delivery of long-term care. *Canadian Medical Association Journal 176*(1), 57–58.

McGregor, M.J., Tate, R.B., McGrail, K.M., Ronald, L.A., Broemeling, A.-M. & Cohen, M. (2006). Care outcomes in long-term care facilities in British Columbia, Canada: Does ownership matter? *Medical Care* 44(10), 929–935.

Moore, D. (2009). Designing long-term care for lesbian, gay, bisexual, transsexual, and transgender people. In P. Armstrong et al. (Eds.), *A place to call home: Long-term care in Canada* (pp. 104–110). Winnipeg: Fernwood Publishing.

National Union of Public and General Employees (NUPGE). (2007). *Dignity denied: Long-term care and Canada's elderly.* Nepean: NUPGE.

Neysmith, S.M. (1997). Towards a woman-friendly long-term care policy. In P. Evans & G. Wekerle (Eds.), *Women and the Canadian welfare state: Challenges and change* (pp. 222–245). Toronto: University of Toronto Press.

Neysmith, S.M. & Aronson, J. (1997). Working conditions in home care: Negotiating race and class boundaries in gendered work. *International Journal of Health Services* 27(3), 479–499.

Ontario Health Coalition (OHC). (2008). *Violence, insufficient care, and downloading of heavy care patients: An evaluation of increasing need and inadequate standards in Ontario's nursing homes.* Toronto: OHC.

Organisation for Economic Co-operation and Development (OECD). (2005). *Long-term care of older people.* Paris: OECD Publishing.

Penning, M.J. & Votova, K. (2009). Aging, health, and health care: From hospital and residential care to home and community care. In B. Singh Bolaria & H.D. Dickinson (Eds.), *Health, illness, and health care in Canada* (4th ed.). 349–369. Toronto: Harcourt Brace.

Pitters, S. (2002). Long-term care facilities. In M. Stephenson & E. Sawyer (Eds.), *Continuing the care: The issues and challenges for long-term care* (pp. 163–202). Ottawa: CHA Press.

Sarma, S., Hawley, G. & Basu, K. (2009). Transitions in living arrangements of Canadian seniors: Findings from the NPHS longitudinal data. *Social Science and Medicine* 68, 1106–1113.

Shapiro, E. & Seeley, M. (2009). Less money, more people: Implications of policy changes in long-term care. In P. Armstrong et al. (Eds.), *A place to call home: Long-term care in Canada* (pp. 58–65). Winnipeg: Fernwood Publishing.

Shapiro, E. & Tate, R.B. (2005). Monitoring the outcomes of quality of care in nursing homes using administrative data. *Canadian Journal on Aging 14,* 755–768.

Statistics Canada. (2007). *A portrait of seniors in Canada 2006* (Catalogue no. 89-519-XIE). Ottawa: Minister of Industry.

Statistics Canada. (2009). *Income in Canada 2007* (Catalogue no. 75-202-X). Ottawa: Minister of Industry.

Statistics Canada. (2010). *Residential care facilities 2007/2008* (Catalogue no. 83-237-X). Ottawa: Minister of Industry.

Stinson, J. (2006). The impact of privatization on women. *Canadian Dimension 40*(3), 27–32.

Volunteer Canada. (2009). *Baby boomers — Your new volunteers.* Ottawa: Volunteer Canada.

Voyer, P., Verreault, R., Mengue, P. & Azizah, G. (2007). Prevalence of falls with minor and major injuries and their associated factors among older adults in long-term care facilities. *International Journal of Older People Nursing 2,* 119–130.

Weeks, L.E., Profit, S., Campbell, B., Graham, H., Chircop, A. & Sheppard-LeMoine, D. (2008). Participation in physical activity: Influences reported by seniors in the community and in long-term care facilities. *Journal of Gerontological Nursing 34*(7), 36–43.

Williams, A. & Crooks, V.A. (2008). Introduction: Space, place, and the geographies of women's caregiving work. *Gender, Place, and Culture, 15*(3), 243–247.

CHAPTER 6

# Caring at Home in Canada

BARBARA CLOW AND KRISTI KEMP

## Introduction

The landscape of home care in Canada is complex. The term refers to care that is provided in homes, but it is also used to denote services that are provided outside of institutional settings, but not necessarily in homes. In some parts of the country, home care is publicly funded and widely accessible, while in other places it is available only to those who can pay for it or to those who can demonstrate that they are utterly *unable* to pay for it. Services may be restricted to medical care or they may involve personal care, household chores, social and emotional support, and the navigation of care. Home care often consists of unpaid work provided by families, charities, and volunteers, but it can also be provided by paid workers who are employees of governments, not-for-profit agencies, or private-sector companies.

Despite the diversity of meanings and models attached to the term "caring in the home," whether paid or unpaid, it is largely women's work. Research has not only demonstrated that women do most of the caring at home, it has also revealed that this work, while often rewarding, can also take a toll on the health and well-being of female caregivers. Women may experience greater care-giver strain—both physical and mental—than men because the care they provide tends to be more demanding in a variety of ways. But it is also the case that women are more likely than men to experience poverty or economic insecurity as a result of caring at home.

Attention to caregiving and to women's caring work has pro-duced a wealth of knowledge, but there are still many gaps in our understanding of what caring at home means to and for different groups of women. New research is shedding light on the experi-ences of visible minority women, lesbians, women with disabili-ties, and immigrant women, but much more remains to be done. At the same time, research on women and caregiving has not necessarily led to policies or programs that address the gendered nature of caring at home. There is consequently a pressing need for research that applies sex- and gender-based analysis to exist-ing policy and program frameworks, and for strategies to trans-late established and emerging knowledge into services that are responsive to the needs of those providing the majority of home care—women.

This chapter begins with an overview of the research, policies, and programs that emerged from some of the most intense years of health care reform in Canada. We summarize what was learned about women's experiences of caring at home, and review policy and program responses. The remainder of the discussion focuses on more recently generated knowledge, policies, and programs. Throughout the chapter, we examine the role of sex and gender: how these determinants shape choices about the provision of care, experiences of caring at home, and the needs of caregivers. Sex- and gender-based analysis enables us to assess whether or not newer policies and programs are designed with women in mind. Our objective is to map the caregiving landscape in Canada: who cares and why, what they need, and what they get or don't get to support the work of caring at home.

# Background

Home care and unpaid caregiving have loomed large in public and political discussions and on research agendas since at least the early 1990s (Canadian Caregiver Coalition, 2000; Canadian Policy Research Networks [CPRN], 2005) not because they are new, but because advances in medical care and reforms to the health care system have created a greater demand for home care services and altered the character and intensity of the work (Armstrong & Kits, 2004). Hospital closures and other cost-cutting measures in the 1980s and 1990s, in combination with new medical technologies, meant that patients were sent home "quicker and sicker" from acute care facilities or were not sent into institutions at all (Women and Health Care Reform, 2002). As a result, more care and more technically sophisticated care, such as chemotherapy and colostomy management, had to be provided in the home by paid and unpaid caregivers (Morris, 2004). The work of caring in the home thus became more common, more demanding, and, ultimately, more crucial to the economic sustainability of publicly funded health care (Armstrong & Armstrong, 2001; Canadian Healthcare Association [CHA], 2009; Hollander, Liu & Chappell, 2009).

Although there has long been—and continues to be—a tendency to refer to "families" as the traditional and appropriate caregivers for children and dependent adults, in fact caring in the home is overwhelmingly the work of women, whether they are paid or unpaid (Morris, 2004; Grant et al., 2004). Some have argued that women are natural nurturers and therefore the most logical choice as caregivers, but as Armstrong and Armstrong (2001) maintain, there is little that is "natural" about women's caring work and, indeed, there is often little choice involved. Gendered assumptions about women's and men's roles, which are embedded in cultures, societies, and families, are often responsible for making caring at home women's work (Armstrong & Armstrong, 2001). Despite the predominance of women in home care, they were largely invisible during the most intense period of health care reform. As Morris observed, "Unbelievably, [women] are still not a part of main-stream research or policy consciousness" (quoted in Pederson & Beattie-Huggan, 2001). The persistent lack of attention to home care as a women's issue led Women and Health Care Reform to convene a meeting of researchers, decision-makers, community organizations, and caregivers in Charlottetown, PEI, in 2001. The workshop helped to raise awareness about the gendered nature of caregiving and fostered discussions about the rights of those who give and receive care in Canada (Pederson & Beattie-Huggan, 2001).

## Women and Home Care

Whether or not women choose to care, there is ample evidence that caregiving can undermine their health and well-being (Gahagan et al., 2004; MacDonald, Phipps & Lethbridge, 2005; Keefe, Hawkins & Fancy, 2006; Beagan et al., 2006; Grant et al., 2004). Compared to male caregivers, female caregivers are more likely to experience poor physical health, disrupted sleep, stress, and decreased social well-being (Keefe, Hawkins & Fancey, 2006). The greater strain women experience as caregivers may be related, in part, to the kinds of duties they perform. Male relatives and neighbours are more likely to undertake work that is episodic and public, such as yardwork, snow removal, and transporting care recipients to medical and other appointments, while female caregivers are more often engaged in work that is intimate and continuous, such as bathing and toileting, or technically demanding, such as wound management and catheter care (Grant et al., 2004; Keefe, Hawkins & Fancy, 2006). Another source of strain for many women is the challenge of balancing the demands of caregiving with those of paid employment (Morris, 2004; MacDonald, Phipps & Lethbridge, 2005). Economic considerations also create added stress and privation for women caring at home. Women who work in the home care sector are generally poorly paid and precariously employed, leaving them without stable, adequate incomes. Women who are trying to balance work and unpaid caregiving responsibilities are also more likely to be in precarious employment, making it difficult to negotiate time off. Research further demonstrates that women are more likely than men to take part-time jobs, to take time off from work, or to take early retirement, all of which can jeopardize their immediate and long-term economic prospects (Morris, 2004; Vézina & Turcotte, 2010; Duxbury et al., 2009). Although many people describe the rewards of caregiving, the strains of doing so undoubtedly fall more heavily on the shoulders of women than men (Gahagan et al., 2004; MacDonald, Phipps & Lethbridge, 2005).

While government restructuring of health care during the 1980s and 1990s—in the name of efficiency and fiscal responsibility— accelerated the need for and dependence on home care, it was not balanced by the development of policies and programs aimed at supporting those who provide care at home, paid or unpaid. Some of the provinces already had publicly funded home care in place and several more introduced it during this period, but often these programs were restricted to particular populations (such as those 65 years of age or older), they were subject to means testing, or they covered only some of the services needed by care recipients, leaving families and individuals to go without care unless they could pay for it themselves (Canadian Healthcare Association, 2009). In some cases, the programs were also vulnerable to political change. For example, "three successive majority governments in Ontario ... took different approaches to reforming home care between 1985 and 1996, each government changing the reforms undertaken by the previous one" (Canadian Healthcare Association, 2009, 25). The federal, provincial, and territorial governments undertook a variety of initiatives on home care, including the creation of the First Nations and Inuit Home and Community Care program in 1999 (Health Canada, 2004), the introduction of a Home Care Reporting System in 2001, and the development of a First Ministers' Accord on Health Care Renewal in 2003, which included commitments to the provision of publicly funded home care. But few, if any, of these efforts acknowledged that women were the backbone of home care programs in Canada.

During the same period, limited policy attention was paid to the needs of unpaid caregivers. The Commission on the Future of Health Care released its final report in 2002, acknowledging the critical role played by "informal" caregivers and even noting that the burden of caregiving was falling especially heavily on the shoulders of women (Commission on the Future of Health Care in Canada, 2002, 184). Commissioner Roy Romanow urged the government to amend the *Canada Health Act* to include home care services. He also recommended that other programs be put in place to support unpaid caregivers, including the possibilities of direct remuneration, tax breaks, job protection, caregiver leave, and respite. In a lengthy commentary on the Romanow Report, Women and Health Care Reform pointed out that the commission had consistently ignored the gendered nature of caring at home. While acknowledging the importance of developing programs to support caregivers, they cautioned against tying these supports to the Employment Insurance (EI) program on the grounds that this approach "would not benefit all women equally" (National Coordinating Group on Health Care Reform and Women, 2003, 36). Despite these kinds of warnings, in 2004, the Compassionate Care Benefit was introduced by the federal government as part of the EI program. The benefit was designed to allow employees who were eligible for EI to take insured leave from their jobs to care for dying loved ones (Joseph et al., 2007; Service Canada, 2010; Stadnyk et al., 2009; Williams et al., 2010). While the policy may have been well intentioned, the decision to embed it in the EI program was expedient, at best, and almost certainly designed to contain costs. In either case, the policy was developed without regard for the gendered nature of caregiving (Armstrong & O'Grady, 2004). Women caregivers who had never worked outside of the home, or who were in casual, seasonal, or part-time employment, were ineligible for the Compassionate Care Benefit because they were ineligible for EI (Flagler & Dong, 2010; Osborne & Margo, 2005; Williams et al., 2010). Moreover, because women's earnings tend to be lower than those of men, even those who are eligible for the benefit receive lower rates of compensation. Women drawing on EI for other reasons, such as disability or maternity leave, might be required to refund some of the money they had received through the Compassionate Care Benefit. Not surprisingly, the use of this benefit has been much lower than originally expected (Stadnyk et al., 2009; Williams et al., 2010).

## That Was Then, This Is Now

In the years since the introduction of the Compassionate Care Benefit, new research has, in many cases, confirmed what we already knew about who provides care, what kinds of care are provided, and what rewards and challenges are associated with caregiving. As in the past, women continue to provide the majority of caring at home (Duxbury et al., 2009). For example, a study of eldercare in Canada revealed that nearly six in 10 women between the ages of 45 and 64 were providing unpaid care to seniors (Cranswick & Dosman, 2008). Admittedly, some researchers contend that there is a more equal balance in the numbers of male and female caregivers in Canada today than there was a decade ago (Pollara, 2007; Russell, 2007), but this assertion requires further investigation because it is inconsistent with other research. But even if this is the case, it does not mean that caring in the home is more equitably distributed among women and men, nor that women and men experience similar types and levels of satisfaction or strain. Women's experiences of caring in the home continue to be qualitatively different from men's because they remain subject to systemic gender-based inequities (Cohen & Murray, 2007; Duxbury et al., 2009). We still assume that women will provide care and we socialize them to do so; in the absence of viable alternatives, they "choose" to do the work (Duxbury et al., 2009, 42–43). At the same time, they remain responsible for the most demanding caregiving tasks, which creates social, emotional, and physical strains that continue to jeopardize their health and well-being (Chappell & Dujela, 2008; Duxbury et al., 2009; Fancey et al., 2008; Lai, 2010; Henz, 2010). As in the past, women's economic security is more likely than men's to be adversely affected by caring at home. Their participation in the labour force may be compromised by caregiving responsibilities, including "foregone opportunity, unpaid labour, career interruption, time lost from work, financial loss and, especially for women, job loss" (Duxbury et al., 2009, 34; see also Cayleff, 2008; Henz, 2010; Lilly et al., 2007; Multiple Sclerosis Society of Canada [MSSC], 2009; Donner et al., 2008; Ontario Human Rights Commission [OHRC], 2006). Economic privation and financial insecurity continue to pose serious threats to women's health and their ability to care at home. We also see that rural caregivers have access to fewer services and supports than their urban counterparts (Canadian Home Care Association, 2008; Crosato, Ward-Griffin & Liepert, 2007; Goins et al., 2009; Joseph, Leach & Turner, 2007).

At the same time, new avenues of research and novel approaches are broadening our understanding of women's caregiving work, especially among vulnerable and minority populations. Caring at home appears to have many common elements for women from diverse social locations, but research increasingly demonstrates that there are also salient differences in the needs and experiences of subpopulations of women.

## Ethnicity and Cultural Identity

Much of the literature on caregiving has and continues to focus on White women and men or simply to ignore differences of ethnicity and cultural identity (Crosato, Ward-Griffin & Liepert, 2007; Duxbury et al., 2009). In 2004, for example, Prokop and her colleagues could find no research on Aboriginal women's experiences of home care. But there are encouraging signs that researchers and policy-makers are beginning to pay attention to the experiences of caregivers in diverse populations.

Research in Canada reveals that Aboriginal caregivers tend to be caring for people who are younger, on average, than those cared for by non-Aboriginal people, probably because of significantly higher rates of illness and lower life expectancy among Aboriginal peoples in Canada. Approximately one-third of Aboriginal caregivers provide care for two or more people at the same time (Health Canada, 2007). More than 60 percent of Aboriginal women have low-paying jobs, which offer little flexibility for caregiving responsibilities (Parrack & Joseph, 2007), and burnout rates are high (Health Canada, 2007). Like non-Aboriginal caregivers, many of whom describe the rewards of providing care, Aboriginal caregivers in Canada also frame the caregiving role as an honour. In one study of Aboriginal women in geographically isolated communities, participants reported both that caregiving was a privilege bestowed upon them by the elders and an opportunity to fulfill gendered, culturally prescribed roles within their communities (Crosato, Ward-Griffin & Liepert, 2007). Another research project undertaken with Native Americans revealed that the caregiver burden was defined in relation to the community rather than to the person providing care. In other words, the burden of caregiving arose from a lack of family and community supports, rather than from the absence of services for individuals.

While Aboriginal caregiver research offers an important new perspective, it also creates challenges for understanding the needs and experiences of Aboriginal *women* because they are lumped in with male caregivers (Crosato, Ward-Griffin & Liepert, 2007). Furthermore, because many of the newer studies focus on the provision of care to elderly people in rural or remote Aboriginal communities, it may be difficult to gauge the impact of rural isolation and culture, for example, or differentiate between the experiences of those in urban versus rural settings (Crosato, Ward-Griffin & Liepert, 2007; Parrack & Joseph, 2007; Pauktuutit Inuit Women of Canada, 2006).

Another limitation of the new literature is that Aboriginal women are discussed mostly in aggregate, rather than as distinct cultural, geographic, or politically defined populations. For example, many government programs are meant to serve both First Nations and Inuit women, although these populations have different health, home care, and caregiving needs based on such differences as geography, culture, language, histories of colonization, and experiences of disease (Cameron, 2007; Health Canada, 2007).

Research on the caregiving experiences of other ethnic minority groups is also beginning to emerge. Many of these studies confirm that, as in the general population, women comprise the majority of caregivers. Similarly, researchers have demonstrated that women from ethnic minority populations experience significant stress and role strain, and are less likely than women from majority groups to access formal supports and services (Beagan et al., 2006; Lai, 2010; Stewart et al., 2006; Suwal, 2010; Yarry, Stevens & McCallum, 2007). Some studies are beginning to identify distinctive features of caring at home for ethnic minority groups, such as the sharing of responsibility across large networks of people, family and non-family members alike (Lai, 2010; Yarry, Stevens & McCallum, 2007). Unfortunately, much of this research does not pay close attention to gendered expectations of caregiving within diverse cultures or undertake critical examinations of the ways in which ethnicity, gender, and caregiving intersect (Evans-Campbell et al., 2007). For instance, some studies have noted that spousal caregiving is less common among elderly people from minority cultural groups (e.g., African Americans, Latin Americans) than among people from "European American" cultures (Yarry et al., 2007), and that in many cases, daughters and daughters-in-law are expected to step in and fulfill this role (Lai, 2010, Suwal, 2010; Yarry et al., 2007). However, no explanation of why this is so or what it might mean is offered. More work is also needed to better understand experiences of racism, language barriers, and the extent to which formal services and supports may not be culturally appropriate (OHRC, 2006; Stewart et al., 2006; Suwal, 2010).

# Age

Much of the literature on caring at home continues to focus on elder care, perhaps as a function of fears that a crisis in unpaid caregiving and home care is looming because the Canadian population is aging (Canadian Healthcare Association [CHA], 2009; Lilly, Laporte & Coyte, 2010). Statistics suggest that by 2056, 25 percent of the population will be over 65, and 10 percent will be over 80 years of age (Cranswick & Dosman, 2008). As women typically live longer than men, women are most likely to be caregivers and care recipients both (Armstrong & Kits, 2004; Neysmith & Reitsma-Street, 2009). These predictions may or may not be accurate, but they are certainly not new (Armstrong & Armstrong, 2001).

That said, in the past five years, women from "the sandwich generation" have been more prominently featured in the caregiving literature (Duxbury et al., 2009; Riley & Bowen, 2005). As a generation, female baby boomers (born between 1945 and 1960) have been more likely to pursue careers and have children later in life than did their mothers. As a result, many are currently "sandwiched" between the generations, caring for their children and aging parents (Cranswick & Dosman, 2008; Duxbury et al., 2009). In addition, many of these women are employed outside of the home (Cayleff, 2008; Duxbury et al., 2009). In Canada, nearly one in five caregivers are women from the sandwich generation, and they spend close to 40 hours a week in paid employment and another 40 in caregiving activities (Duxbury et al., 2009). In addition to the massive caregiver strain that is likely to develop for these women, they may also be "adversely affected by the competing and compounding demands on their financial resources" (Duxbury et al., 2009).

Another group that is receiving greater attention in the literature on caregiving is youth. According to a literature review conducted for the Young Carers Initiative of Niagara (Ontario), there is a growing number of youth under the age of 18, who care for parents and other family members facing a range of challenges, including chronic health problems, addictions, physical disabilities, mental illness, and language barriers (Baago, 2005). Although there is a dearth of knowledge about young caregivers in Canada, literature from the United Kingdom and the United States suggests that this is a growing phenomenon that needs policy and program responses (Warren, 2006; Charles, Stainton & Marshall, 2009; Gray, Robinson & Seddon, 2008; National Alliance for Caregiving [NAC], 2005). Interestingly, much of the literature reports that equal numbers of girls and boys act as caregivers (Aldridge & Sharpe, 2007; Baago, 2005). While a few studies point to salient gender differences, such as the fact that girls spend more time than boys caring at home, none of them explore the meaning of these differences (NAC, 2005).

## Sexual Orientation and Gender Identity

In general, people from lesbian, gay, bisexual, two-spirited, transgender, intersex, and queer (LGBTIQ) communities continue to be mostly absent from the literature on caregiving (Cayleff, 2008; Cohen & Murray, 2007). The research that does exist tends to focus on LGBTIQ people as care recipients as opposed to providers of care (Brotman, Ryan & Meyer, 2006; MetLife Mature Market Institute [MMMI], 2010), or as caregivers to people with HIV/AIDS (Cohen & Murray, 2007). As with other subpopulations, LGBTIQ caregivers face distinct challenges related to their social location. Female LGBTIQ caregivers, in particular, may be subject to considerable pressure from family to provide care, on the assumption that they are more "available"; in the absence of a male partner, they are assumed to be single even when they have partners and children (Beagan et al., 2006; Cayleff, 2008). Lesbians without children are also likely to be conscripted into care for similar reasons (Beagan et al., 2006; Cohen & Murray, 2007; Cayleff, 2008). Caregivers from the LGBTIQ community often fear homophobia, and may experience intolerance and a lack of support from care recipients (OHRC, 2006). Some studies have begun to explore the complexities of caring for someone who denies or disapproves of the caregiver's sexual orientation or gender identity (Beagan et al., 2006; Cohen & Murray, 2007; Hash & Cramer, 2003). For these women, caregiving can become a particularly isolating experience.

Interestingly, some research is emerging to suggest that within LGBTIQ communities, men are more likely than women to care at home (MMMI, 2010). This is in direct contrast to research findings among those with a heterosexual orientation or in heterodominant contexts. Cohen and Murray (2007) suggest that more fluid and flexible gender roles in LGBTIQ communities may contribute to men feeling more comfortable with caregiving duties traditionally assigned to women. Another notable difference in LGBTIQ communities is that caregiving for friends (also described as "chosen family") is far more common (21 percent) than in non-LGBTIQ communities (6 percent) (see also Cayleff, 2008; Cohen & Murray, 2007; Hash & Cramer, 2003).

## Ability and Disability

Research on disability and caregiving usually focuses on the needs of care recipients (Keefe, Légaré & Carrière, 2007), ignoring the fact that women with disabilities are likely to be care recipients at the same time that they are care providers (Beagan et al., 2006). Caregivers living with disabilities may require more support than other caregivers, depending on the nature of their disability (Gahagan et al., 2004; Martinez, Williams & Fuhr, 2009). They may also experience additional barriers that magnify the stresses associated with caring at home, including a lack of accessible transportation (Gahagan et al., 2004; Lutz & Bowers, 2005), a shortage of caregiver support programs designed for people with disabilities (OHRC, 2006), greater levels of fatigue (Gahagan et al., 2004), and higher levels of isolation (Martinez, Williams & Fuhr,

2009). Further, women with disabilities earn lower wages than other women (DisAbled Women's Network [DAWN] Canada, n.d.; Lutz & Bowers, 2005; OHRC, 2006), and if they are unable to work, must rely on income security programs that "virtually guarantee a life of poverty for many" (Torjman, 2009, 2).

# Location

In addition to new research on diverse populations of women caregivers, there are also interesting new studies about the meaning of "home" and the gendered nature of private space. Armstrong and Kits (2004), among others, have contested the traditional view of the home as a safe space, a natural location for giving and receiving care. Sometimes the space itself is unsuitable for caring for a variety of reasons and, increasingly, unpaid and paid caregivers do not have the skills necessary to provide safe care. But there is also a need to consider the risk and impact of violence and abuse. For example, studies featuring lesbian caregivers of elderly parents revealed that caring for their parents at home meant that they were often forced back into the closet (Beagan et al., 2006; Cayleff, 2008; Hash & Cramer, 2003). In one case, a caregiver found herself obliged to care for a parent who had abused her as a child (Beagan et al., 2006). This is an important and neglected area of research, given that 83 percent of women have experienced violence at the hands of their spouse (Statistics Canada, 2009), and 80 percent of sexual assault victims are girls, with the majority of their perpetrators being family members (Calhoun Research and Development & C. Lang Consulting, 2005; Canadian Centre for Justice Statistics, 2005).

Other researchers are also beginning to reconfigure the idea of home as both public and private space. As Dyck et al. (2005) assert, "Care is provided in spaces designed for other purposes, of varying sizes and conditions, and where there are strong associations with the notions of privacy and 'family life'" (p. 174). Home as the location for unpaid work is not a new phenomenon for women, given that "the home" and much of what it encompasses (children, housework) continue to be considered the female domain (Williams & Crooks, 2008). Although new studies addressing the intersection of gender and home care are few, those that exist are powerful. For example, in a retrospective analysis of interviews with home care workers and the family members who employed them, Martin-Matthews (2007) found a gendered division of spaces within the home. Bathrooms and bedrooms were deemed to be "private" spaces that were accessed mostly by women because male caregivers (sons, sons-in-law) were not expected to undertake the intimate "body work" that occurred in these spaces (Brazil et al., 2009; CHA, 2009; Chappell & Dujela, 2008; Henz, 2010; Martin-Matthews, 2007). Martin-Matthews' study also analyzed the gendered experiences of care recipients related to the care that was provided to them at home. For instance, elderly female care recipients were more likely to be "territorial" about their physical space, especially with female caregivers, whereas men were far less likely be concerned about spatial breaches of privacy and loss of control of private space. Similarly, Dyck and others (2005) commented that bringing caregivers into a home challenges its "privateness" and the identities of the care recipients who live there. For some caregivers and some care recipients, a significant dimension of caring at home may be the experience that one person's abode becomes another's workplace.

## Supporting Caregivers: Policy and Program Initiatives

A review of policy and program initiatives since 2004 reveals some change, but not enough. Governments in Canada—as in other countries—continue to assume that the care of the aged, ill, and disabled will be largely provided by family members with public supports and services created to "fill in the gaps" (Lilly et al., 2007). As in the past, many programs and policies ignore the diversity of families and caregivers, as well as the dynamics and duration of caring at home (Montgomery & Kosloski, 2009). Kershaw, writing about parental leave, asserted that the government should "use public policy to influence men's choices directly so that they select more gender-progressive practices over the patriarchal patterns that intersect with ethnic and class divisions of care to disadvantage diverse groups of women" (p. 343). While it is encouraging to see attention to the gendered nature of policies, programs, and practices, supports for caregivers in Canada are still being designed with little or no attention to the gendered nature of caring at home. The Compassionate Care Benefit, mentioned earlier, is a case in point. In a 2010 evaluation of the CCB program (Williams et al., 2010), caregivers stressed the importance of improving access for diverse groups of women. Caregivers recommended making it more available to those who are self-employed or in part-time jobs, transforming it from an EI benefit to a refundable tax credit, and expanding its scope to include chronic illnesses and disabilities, rather than just palliative situations (Osborne & Margo, 2005; Torjman, 2009).

The federal government has also pursued a number of policies and strategies to enhance primary and home care services for Aboriginal peoples in Canada, including the Aboriginal Health Transition Fund (AHTF). Introduced in 2004, the AHTF funded projects aimed at improving health services for Aboriginal peoples and some of these projects dealt with home care, unpaid caregiving, and palliative care (Health Canada, 2008). Recipients of funding were required to demonstrate gender analyses in their proposals, but as the results and reports of these projects are still pending, it remains to be seen whether or not the work was either gendered or culturally appropriate. As the reports become available, it will be important for researchers and policy-makers to follow up. In 2004, Health Canada also began a series of evaluations of the First Nations Inuit Home and Community Care Program (FNIHCCP) (Health Canada, 2007). Although the program does not focus on informal caregivers or their needs per se, a number of initiatives were related to caring at home, including increasing the cultural competence of nurses and paid home care support workers, making assessment processes for paid home care services more culturally sensitive, and bringing home care services to rural and remote areas (Cameron, 2007; Health Canada, 2004). While this was a promising step on the part of the federal government, the needs of First Nations and Inuit women caregivers were not addressed explicitly within the program, nor were their voices evident in the evaluation process.

Provincial governments have begun to respond to the needs of those caring at home by supporting caregiver networks and organizations, creating respite programs, and offering varying levels of financial assistance and tax breaks. In some provinces—British Columbia, Alberta, Saskatchewan, Quebec, Nova Scotia, and Newfoundland/Labrador—caregiver support organizations are independent of government, but rely on provincial funding to deliver a variety of services, such as telephone hotlines, formalized support networks/groups, and web-based information. The remaining provinces provide support through government agencies and they tend to offer fewer or less well-developed services as evidenced by the limited information on websites. The governments of the Yukon, the Northwest Territories, and Nunavut offer even fewer resources for caregivers. In an effort to address some of the financial inequities caregivers experience, three provinces have recently created benefits or tax credits for those providing unpaid care. In 2008, Manitoba introduced a primary caregiver tax credit of $1,020 per year for caregivers (Manitoba Health, 2008) and in 2009, passed a home care service policy that provides remuneration for family members providing non-professional home care services (Manitoba Health, 2009). In 2009, Nova Scotia created an allowance of up to $400 per month for caregivers providing more than 20 hours of care per week to an individual with significant care needs (Government of Nova Scotia, 2009). Quebec is the only province to offer a tax credit for respite services, as well as a tax credit for caregivers (Revenu Québec, 2009). While many of these initiatives are promising, they generally do not acknowledge that women are the majority of those who provide care at home, and most program and services are not tailored to the needs of women.

# Conclusion

Care at home, provided by women, often at no charge, is a critical component of health care in Canada and it deserves greater recognition, compensation, and support. This is something we have known for a long time. The presentations featured at the 2001 workshop on home care, hosted by Women and Health Care Reform—and the discussions that arose from those presentations—underscored the imperative of addressing women's experiences and needs as caregivers. As the organizers concluded, "We agreed that, while there remain critical gaps in research, there is enough research to provide a basis for action. From the opening session … there is a sense among us that part of what had to happen over the course of our meeting was to find a way to articulate the urgent need for action, for both care providers and those who receive care" (Pederson & Beattie-Huggan, 2001). A framework for action, *The Charlottetown Declaration on the Right to Care*, emerged from the workshop, outlining the principles for a national health care system that includes home care and the women who provide it (see Appendix).

Unfortunately, as we have seen in this discussion, the gendered nature of caregiving and home care still remains unacknowledged by many researchers, organizations, and governments. As the Canadian population ages, and more women become care recipients and caregivers alike, it will become increasingly necessary to include analyses of sex and gender, as well as their intersections with age, ethnicity, culture, ability, and other determinants of health if we hope to create supports and policies that are useful and appropriate. Indeed, as we learn more about caregivers in non-dominant cultures and begin to approach the study of caregiving in new ways, this need becomes more apparent and compelling.

# References

Aldridge, J. & Sharpe, D. (2007). *Pictures of young caring*. Retrieved from http://www.lboro.ac.uk/departments/ss/centres/YCRG/youngCarers-Download/Pictures%20of%20young%20caring%20research%20 report.pdf

Armstrong, P. & Armstrong, H. (2001). Thinking it through: Women, work, and caring in the new millennium. Retrieved from http:// www.acewh.dal.ca/eng/reports/Thinking-It-Through-web.pdf

Armstrong, P. & Kits, O. (2004). One hundred years of caregiving. In K.R. Grant, C. Amaratunga, P. Armstrong, M. Boscoe, A. Pederson & K. Wilson (Eds.), *Caring for/ caring about: Women, home care, and unpaid caregiving* (pp. 45–73). Aurora: Garamond Press.

Armstrong, P. & O'Grady, P. (2004). *Compassionate care benefits not compassionate enough*. Retrieved from http://www.cwhn.ca/resources/ kickers/homecare.html

Baago, S. (2005). *Inside the "developmental black box" of young carers*. Retrieved from http://www.youngcarers.ca/articles/BlackboxAu-gust2007.pdf

Beagan, B., Stadnyk, R., Loppie, C., MacDonald, N., Hamilton-Hinch, B. & MacDonald, J. (2006). *Snapshots of the lives of caregivers: Caregiver portraits. "I do it because I love her and I care."* Retrieved from http://www.acewh.dal.ca/eng/reports/TeamP-Report-web.pdf

Brazil, K., Thabane, L., Foster, G. & Bédard, M. (2009). Gender differences among Canadian spousal caregivers at the end of life. *Health and Social Care in the Community 17(2),* 159–166.

Brotman, S., Ryan, B. & Meyer, E. (2006). *The health and social service needs of gay and lesbian seniors and their families in Canada*. Retrieved from http://www.mcgill.ca/files/interaction/Executive_Summary.pdf

Calhoun Research and Development & C. Lang Consulting. (2005).

*Girls in Canada 2005: A report prepared for the Canadian Women's Foundation.* Retrieved from http://www.cdnwomen.org/PDFs/EN/ CWF-GirlsCanada-Report05.pdf

Cameron, E. (2007). *State of the knowledge: Inuit public health.* Retrieved from http://www.kamatsiaqtut.com/images/Inuit_Public_Health,Final_ Report_Apr_26_2007.pdf

Canadian Caregiver Coalition. (2000). *Report of the proceedings of the founding meeting.* Retrieved from http://www.ccc-ccan.ca/media. php?mid=57

Canadian Caregiver Coalition. (2008a). *Caregiver facts.* Retrieved from http://www.ccc-can.ca/ media.php?mid=124

Canadian Caregiver Coalition. (2008b). *A framework for a Canadian caregiver strategy.* Retrieved from http://www.ccc-ccan.ca/media. php?mid=229

Canadian Centre for Justice Statistics. (2005). *Family violence in Canada: A statistical profile.* Retrieved from http://www.statcan.gc.ca/ pub/85-224-x/85-224-x2005000-eng.pdf

Canadian Healthcare Association [CHA]. (2009). *Home care in Canada: From the margins to the mainstream.* Ottawa: CHA. Retrieved from http://www.chalearning.ca/documents/ Home_Care_in_Canada_ From_the_ Margins_to_the_Mainstream_web.pdf

Canadian Home Care Association. (2008). *A scan of options for delivering home care in rural, remote, and northern regions of Canada.* Retrieved from http://www.cdnhomecare.ca/ media.php?mid=2174

Canadian Institute of Health Information. (2010). *Supporting informal caregivers: The heart of home care.* Retrieved from http://www.secure. cihi.ca/cihiweb/products/ Caregiver_Distress_AIB_2010_EN.pdf

Canadian Policy Research Networks (CPRN). (2005). *A healthy balance: Caregiving policy in Canada—backgrounder.* Retrieved from http:// www.cprn.org/documents/40910_en.pdf

Cayleff, S. (2008). Feeding the hand that bit you: Lesbian daughters at mid-life negotiating parental caretaking. *Journal of Lesbian Studies* 12(2–3), 237–254.

Chappell, N.L. & Dujela, C. (2008). Caregiving: Predicting at-risk status. *Canadian Journal on Aging* 27(2), 169–179.

Charles, G., Stainton, T. & Marshall, S. (2009). Young carers: Mature before their time. *Reclaiming Children and Youth 8*(2), 38–41.

Cohen, H.L. & Murray, Y. (2007). Chapter 14: Older lesbian and gay caregivers. *Journal of Human Behavior in the Social Environment 14*(1), 275–298.

Commission on the Future of Health Care in Canada. (2002). *Building on values: The future of health care in Canada.* Ottawa: Government of Canada.

Cranswick, K. & Dosman, D. (2008). Eldercare: What we know today. *Canadian Social Trends*, 47–57. Statistics Canada. Volume 89 (Catalogue no. 11-008). Retrieved from http://www.statcan.gc.ca.libaccess.lib. mcmaster.ca/pub/11-008-x/2008002/article/10689-eng.pdf

Crosato, K.E., Ward-Griffin, C. & Leipert, B. (2007). Aboriginal women caregivers of the elderly in geographically isolated communities. *Rural and Remote Health 7.* Retrieved from http://www.rrh.org.au/publishedarticles/article_print_796.pdf

DisAbled Women's Network [DAWN]. (n.d.). Retrieved from http://www.dawncanada.net/pdf/ StudyonEconomicSecurityonWomenwithDisabilitiesEng.pdf

Donner, L., Isfeld, H., Haworth-Brockman, M. & Forsey, C. (2008). *A profile of women's health in Manitoba.* Winnipeg: Prairie Women's Health Centre of Excellence. Retrieved from http://www.pwhce.ca/profile/pdf/ProfileWomensHealthManitoba Complete.pdf

Dunbrack, J. (2007). *The policy implications of 13 caregiver respite projects.* Retrieved from http://www.mcconnellfoundation.ca/assets/Media%20Library/Reports/Care%20Renewal%20The%20policy%20implications%20of%2013%20caregiver%20respite%20projects. pdf

Duxbury, L., Higgins, C. & Schroeder, B. (2009). *Balancing paid work and caregiving responsibilities: A close look at family caregivers in Canada.* Retrieved from http://www.cprn.org/documents/51061_EN.pdf

Dyck, I., Kontos, P., Angus, J. & McKeever, P. (2005). The home as a site for long-term care: Meanings and management of bodies and space. *Health & Place 11*, 173–185.

Evans-Campbell, T., Fredriksen-Goldsen, K.I., Walters, K.L. & Stately, A. (2007). Caregiving experiences among American Indian twospirit men and women: Contemporary and historical roles. *Journal of Gay and Lesbian Social Services 18*(3–4), 75–92.

Fancey, P., Keefe, J., Guberman, N. & Barylak, L. (2008). *The C.A.R.E. tool: Examining the role of caregiver assessment in health promotion of older spousal caregivers.* Retrieved from http://www.msvu.ca/site/media/msvu/PHAC%20older%20spousal%20 caregiving_paper_Mar_31%20FINAL.pdf

Flagler, J. & Dong, W. (2010). The uncompassionate elements of the Compassionate Care Benefits program: A critical analysis. *Global Health Promotion 17*(1), 50–59.

Gahagan, J., Loppie, C., MacLellan, M., Rehman, L. & Side, K. (2004). *Caregiver resilience and the quest for balance: A report on findings from focus groups.* Halifax: Healthy Balance Research Program. Retrieved from http://www.acewh.dal.ca/eng/reports/ TeamQ-web.pdf

Gamble, B.J. (2009). Canadian stakeholders' views about the boundaries of publicly funded health care: What are the consequences for women caregivers? *Women's Health and Urban Life 6*(2), 22–35.

Goins, R.T., Spencer, S.M. & Byrd, J.C. (2009). Research on rural caregiving: A literature review. *Journal of Applied Gerontology 28*(2), 139–170.

Government of Nova Scotia. (2009, November). *The caregiver allowance.* Retrieved from http://www.gov.ns.ca/health/ccs/caregiver_allowance.asp

Grant, K.R., Amaratunga, C., Armstrong, P., Boscoe, M., Pederson, A. & Willson, K. (2004). *Caring for/caring about: Women, home care, and unpaid caregiving.* Aurora: Garamond.

Gray, B., Robinson, C. & Seddon, D. (2008). Invisible children: Young carers of parents with mental health problems. *Child and Adolescent Mental Health 13*(4), 169–172.

Hash, K.M. & Cramer, E.P. (2003). Empowering gay and lesbian caregivers and uncovering their unique experiences through the use of qualitative methods. *Journal of Gay and Lesbian Social Services 15*(1/2), 47–63.

Health Canada. (2004, December). *First Nations and Inuit Home and Community Care Program (FNIHCCP): Study 1, implementation "foundations for success" summary report: Executive summary and key findings.* Retrieved from http://www.hc-sc.gc.ca/fniah-spnia/alt_formats/

fnihb-dgspni/pdf/pubs/home-domicile/2004_foundat-fondat_success-eng.pdf

Health Canada. (2007). *First Nations and Inuit health program compendium.* Retrieved from http://www.hc-sc.gc.ca/fniah-spnia/alt_formats/fnihb-dgspni/pdf/pubs/gen/cs-133_compendium-eng.pdf

Health Canada. (2008). *Aboriginal Health Transition Fund (AHTF)— $7.6M for eight Inuit-specific projects.* Retrieved from http://www.hc-sc.gc.ca/ahc-asc/media/nr-cp/_2008/2008_09bk1-eng.php

Henz, U. (2010). Parent care as unpaid family labor: How do spouses share? *Journal of Marriage and Family 72,* 148–164.

Hollander, M.J., Liu, G. & Chappell, N.L. (2009). Who cares and how much? The imputed economic contribution to the Canadian healthcare system of middle-aged and older unpaid caregivers providing care to the elderly. *Healthcare Quarterly 12*(2), 42–49.

Joseph, G., Leach, B. & Turner, S. (2007). *Caring at a distance: Working women, rural to urban migration, and the compassionate care challenge.* Guelph: Centre for Family, Work, and Wellbeing.

Keefe, J., Hawkins, G. & Fancey, P. (2006). *A portrait of unpaid care in Nova Scotia.* Retrieved from http://www.acewh.dal.ca/eng/reports/Portrait-of-Unpaid-Care-web.pdf

Keefe, J., Légaré, J. & Carrière, Y. (2007). Developing new strategies to support caregivers of older Canadians with disabilities: Projections of need and their policy implications. *Canadian Public Policy 33*(Supplement), S66–S80.

Keefe, J.M., Fancey, P. & White, S. (2005). *Consultation on financial compensation initiatives for family caregivers of dependent adults.* Halifax: Maritime Data Centre for Aging Research and Policy Analysis, Mount Saint Vincent University.

Keefe, J.M. & Manning, M. (2005). *The cost effectiveness of respite: A literature review.* Retrieved from http://www.hc-sc.gc.ca/hcs-sss/alt_formats/hpb-dgps/pdf/pubs/2005-keefe/2005 keefe-eng.pdf

Kershaw, P.W. (2006). Carefair: Choice, duty, and the distribution of care. *Social Politics: International Studies in Gender, State, and Society 13*(3), 341–371.

Kim, Y. & Schulz, R. (2008). Family caregivers' strains: Comparative analysis of cancer caregiving with dementia, diabetes, and frail elderly caregiving. *Journal of Aging and Health 20*(5), 483–503.

Krogh, K. (2004). Redefining home care for women with disabilities: A call for citizenship. In K.R. Grant, C. Amaratunga, P. Armstrong, M. Boscoe, A. Pederson & K. Wilson (Eds.), *Caring for/caring about: Women, home care, and unpaid caregiving* (pp. 115–146). Aurora: Garamond Press.

Lai, D.W.L. (2010). Filial piety, caregiving appraisal, and caregiving burden. *Research on Aging 32*(2), 200–223.

Lilly, M.B., Laporte, A. & Coyte, P.C. (2007). Labor market work and home care's unpaid caregivers: A systematic review of labor force participation rates, predictors of labor market withdrawal, and hours of work. *The Milbank Quarterly 85*(4), 641–690.

Lilly, M.B., Laporte, A. & Coyte, P.C. (2010). Do they care too much to work? The influence of caregiving intensity on the labour force participation of unpaid caregivers in Canada. *Journal of Health Economics 29*, 895–903.

Lutz, B.J. & Bowers, B.J. (2005). Disability in everyday life. *Qualitative Health Research 15*(8), 1037–1054.

MacDonald, M., Phipps, S. & Lethbridge, L. (2005). Taking its toll: The influence of paid and unpaid work on women's well-being. *Feminist Economics 11*, 63–94.

Manitoba Health. (2008). *Manitoba home care program: Primary caregiver tax credit.* Retrieved from wwwgov.mb.ca/health/homecare/pctc.html

Manitoba Health. (2009). *Manitoba home care program: Engagement of family members to provide non-professional home care services.* Retrieved from www.gov.mb.ca/health/homecare/nonprof.html.

Martinez, B.S., Williams, M. & Fuhr, P. (2009). Visually impaired caregivers: Perspectives from patient focus groups. *Optometry 80*(1), 11–22.

Martin-Matthews, A. (2007). Situating "home" at the nexus of the public and private spheres: Ageing, gender, and home support work in Canada. *Current Sociology 55*(2), 229–249.

MetLife Mature Market Institute [MMMI]. (2010). *Still out, still aging: The MetLife study of lesbian, gay, bisexual, and transgender baby boomers.* Retrieved from http://www.metlife. com/assets/cao/mmi/

publications/studies/2010/mmi-still-out-still-aging.pdf

Miller, E.A., Allen, S.M. & Mor, V. (2009). Commentary: Navigating the labyrinth of long-term care: Shoring up informal caregiving in a home- and community-based world. *Journal of Aging & Social Policy 21*, 1–16.

Montgomery, J. V. & Kosloski, K. (2009). Caregiving as a process of changing identity: Implications for caregiver support. *Generations 33*(1), 47–52.

Morris, M. (2004). What research reveals about gender, home care, and caregiving: Overview and the case for gender analysis. In K.R. Grant, C. Amaratunga, P. Armstrong, M. Boscoe, A. Pederson & K. Wilson (Eds.), *Caring for/caring about: Women, home care, and unpaid caregiving* (pp. 91–113). Aurora: Garamond Press.

Multiple Sclerosis Society of Canada [MSSC]. (2009). *Caregiver and poverty stakeholder forum: Summary report.* Retrieved from http://www. mssociety.ca/en/pdf/pub_C&PFinalReport.pdf

National Alliance for Caregiving [NAC]. (2005). *Young carers in the US.* Retrieved from http://www.caregiving.org/data/youngcaregivers. pdf

National Coordinating Group on Health Care Reform and Women. (2003). *Reading Romanow: The implications of the final report of the Commission on the Future of Health Care in Canada for women.* Toronto: National Coordinating Group on Health Care Reform and Women.

Neysmith, S.M. & Reitsma-Street, M. (2009). The provisioning responsibilities of older women. *Journal of Aging Studies 23*(4), 236–244.

Ontario Human Rights Commission [OHRC]. (2006). *The cost of caring.* Retrieved from http://www.ohrc.on.ca/en/ resources/ discussion_consultation/famconsult/pdf

Osborne, K. & Margo, N. (2005). *Analysis and evaluation: Compassionate Care Benefit.* Retrieved from http://www.healthcouncilcanada.ca/ docs/papers/2005/ Compassionate_Care_BenefitsEN.pdf

Parrack, S. & Joseph, G.M. (2007). The informal caregivers of Aboriginal seniors: Perspectives and issues. *First People's Child and Family Review 3*(4), 106–113.

Pauktuutit Inuit Women of Canada. (2006). *Urban Inuit family caregivers workshop: Contributions and concerns*. Retrieved from http://www. pauktuutit.ca/caregivers/ downloads/Concerns.pdf

Pederson, A. & P. Beattie-Huggan (2001). *The objective is care: Proceedings of the national think tank on gender and unpaid caregiving*. Retrieved from http://www.womenandhealthcarereform.ca/publications/ guc-think-tanken.pdf

Peters, H., Fiske, J., Hemingway, D., Vaillancourt, A., McLennan, C., Keith, B. & Burrill, A. (2010). Interweaving caring and economics in the context of place: Experiences of northern and rural women caregivers. *Ethics and Social Welfare* 4(2), 172–187.

Pollara (2007). *The 10th annual health care in Canada survey*. Retrieved from http://www.hcic-sssc.ca/english/files/CurrentContent/2007/2007_ hcic.pdf

Professionals Networking for Caregivers website. (2008). Retrieved from http://www.rppa-pnc.com

Prokop, S.T., Haug, E., Hogan, M., McCarthy, J. & MacDonald, L. (2004). Aboriginal women and home care. In K.R. Grant, C. Amaratunga, P. Armstrong, M. Boscoe, A. Pederson, & K. Willson (Eds.), *Caring for/caring about: Women, home care, and unpaid caregiving* (pp. 147–166). Aurora: Garamond Press.

Rajnovich, B., Keefe, J. & Fast, J. (2005). *Supporting caregivers of dependent adults in the 21st century*. Retrieved from http://www.acewh.dal.ca/ eng/reports/Supporting _caregivers_of_dependent_Adults.pdf

Revenu Québec. (2009, November.) *Informal caregivers*. Retrieved from http://www.revenu.gouv. qc.ca/en/citoyen/clientele/aidant/ default.aspx

Riley, L.D. & Bowen, C.P. (2005). The sandwich generation: Challenges and coping strategies of multigenerational families. *The Family Journal: Counseling and Therapy for Couples and Families* 13(1), 52–58.

Russell, R. (2007). Men doing "women's work": Elderly men caregivers and the gendered construction of care work. *The Journal of Men's Studies* 15(1), 1–18.

Senate Special Committee on Aging. (2009). *Canada's aging population: Seizing the opportunity*. Retrieved from http://www.senate-senat.ca/ age.asp

Service Canada. (2010). *Compassionate care benefits*. Retrieved from http://

www.servicecanada.gc.ca/eng/ei/types/compassionate_care.shtml

Stadnyk, R., Fletcher, S., Eales, J., Fast, J. & Keating, N. (2009). *Employed family/friend caregivers to adults with disabilities: The impact of public policies on caregivers' costs*. Retrieved from http://www.uofaweb. ualberta.ca/hcic/pdfs/HCIC_Impact_ of_public_policies_on_caregivers%27_costs_final_report_09May20_%282%29.pdf

Statistics Canada. (2009). *Family violence in Canada: A statistical profile*. Retrieved from http://www.dsp-psd.pwgsc.gc.ca/collection_2009/statcan/85-224-X/85-224-x2009000-eng.pdf

Stewart, M.J., Neufeld, A., Harrison, M.J., Spitzer, D., Hughes, K. & Makwarimba, E. (2006). Immigrant women family caregivers in Canada: Implications for policies and programmes in health and social sectors. *Health and Social Care in the Community* 14(4), 329–340.

Suwal, J.V. (2010). Health consequences to immigrant family caregivers in Canada. *Canadian Studies in Population* 37(1–2), 107–124.

Torjman, S. (2009). *Caledon commentary: The three ghosts of poverty*. Retrieved from http://www.caledoninst.org/Publications/PDF/831ENG.pdf

Vézina, M. & Turcotte, M. (2010). Caring for a parent who lives far away: The consequences. *Canadian Social Trends*. Statistics Canada. Volume 89 (Catalogue no. 11-008).

Warren, J. (2006). Young carers: Conventional or exaggerated levels of involvement in domestic and caring tasks? *Children & Society* 21(2): 136–146.

Williams, A. & Crooks, V.A. (2008). Introduction: Space, place, and the geographies of women's caregiving work. *Gender, Place & Culture* 15(3), 243–247.

Williams, A., Crooks, V.A., Giesbrecht, M. & Dykeman, S. (2010). *Evaluating Canada's Compassionate Care Benefit from the perspective of family caregivers*. Retrieved from http://www.ccc-ccan.ca/media.php?mid=287

Women and Health Care Reform. (2002). *Women and home care: Why does home care matter to women?* Retrieved from http://www.womenandhealthcarereform.ca/publications/why-hc-matter.pdf

Yarry, S.J., Stevens, E.K. & McCallum, T.J. (2007). Cultural influences on spousal caregiving. *Generations* 31(3), 24–30.

CHAPTER 7

# Women's Work in Health Care

PAT ARMSTRONG

Access to health care and its quality are profoundly shaped by the organization of work in health services. Given that more than 80 percent of those employed in health and social care are women (Canadian Institute for Health Information [CIHI], 2007), and that women account for the majority both of those providing unpaid personal care (Zukewich, 2003) and of those using the health care services, work organization in health care is clearly an issue for women. But numbers alone fail to capture the range of issues for women as care providers and as those with care needs. Given the important differences among women as both providers and patients, numbers also fail to identify the problems faced by particular groups of women.

This chapter focuses on the division of labour in health care work. It explores the major occupations in health and social care to identify significant issues for women as a group and for women in different social, physical, and geographical locations. Space does not allow for a detailed analysis of all the work in care or of differences among women. The purpose here is to demonstrate the need for a gender-based analysis through an overview of occupations in health care, highlighting some critical ways in which gender is implicated. In keeping with our practice of seeking to make visible the invisible in women's health, Women and Health Care Reform has focused on those usually described as ancillary, namely, those who cook, clean, do laundry and clerical work, and those who provide personal care. This chapter begins with doctors and nurses, however, for two reasons. First, as in other chapters, our purpose is to move beyond our previous work to provide an overview of gender issues for women and thus it is necessary to include those who make up such a significant and powerful part of this labour force. Second, although doctors and nurses are the ones most frequently considered in discussion of "health human resources," the kind of gender analysis we undertake is often absent in these discussions.

## Doctors

The Canadian health care system is organized to have doctors as the primary gatekeepers. As a result, the number of doctors, their sex, their location, and their approaches to care are critical factors in women's access to health services. In addition, the ways in which medicine is taught, organized, and funded have a significant impact on women physicians, on other health care workers, and on their patients. This section highlights some of the implications of these factors for women as patients, as well as for the growing number of women who work in medicine.

Gender-based analysis is seldom part of official reports on health care providers. Gender has, however, received considerable attention in the discussion of doctor supply. Some of this attention can be explained by the dramatic increase in the number of women practising medicine, in contrast to the long-standing numerical dominance of women throughout the rest of health services. According to the Canadian Institute for Health Information (CIHI, 2009b, Data Table 1.1), in 2008, 56 percent of family physicians younger than 40 were women, compared to 16 percent of family physicians 60 and older. Still only a third of practising physicians, women are set to become the majority before long.

But numbers alone do not explain the focus on gender in discussions of doctors. Some of the explanation can be found in mass media publicity and journal articles about concerns over how women practise medicine and what this means in terms of access. A 2008 *Maclean's* article began with an anecdote about a woman doctor leaving her job to be with her family and quoted health economist Peter Coyte as saying that "this influx of women will contribute to the crisis in health care" (Gulli & Lunau, 2008, 23). The article prompted an editorial in the *Canadian Medical Association Journal* titled "Ending the Sexist Blame Game," in which the authors argued that the "decline in physicians' working hours is attributed more to the decline in hours worked by male physicians than the increasing proportion of female physicians" (Herbert, Whiteside, McKnight, Verma & Wilson, 2008, 659). A year later, a *National Post* headline declared that "Female doctors hurt productivity" (Blackwell, 2009), citing a study that claimed women doctors worked fewer hours providing direct patient care and saw fewer patients during those hours, in addition to taking more family leaves (Weizblit, Noble & Baerlocher, 2009). Yet in the same news story the president of the Canadian Medical Association cautioned that younger doctors practise medicine differently than older ones, spending more time with patients and placing more emphasis on family, so we have to be careful about attributing change to gender alone (Blackwell, 2009). It is also important to note that hours of work are not the only factors influencing supply. For example, male physicians were more likely than their female counterparts to take jobs abroad (CIHI, 2008, tables 14.1, 14.2).

Equally important, the fact that women often practise medicine differently than men could well be seen as an improvement in medicine and in women's access to health care rather than as a problem for care. The study that prompted the media coverage of women doctors' hours (Weizblit et al., 2009) also points out that women specialists are more likely to work in pediatrics, obstetrics, and gynecology than men. They are also more likely to work in family practices and primary care. Thus, the influx of women means greater access to many of the services women are most likely to use. Moreover, the research also suggests that women spend more time with each patient, promote more open and equal exchange with patients (Roter, Hall & Aoki, 2002), are more likely to counsel patients about condom use (Maheux, Haley, Rivard & Gervais, 1997), and are more likely both to address mental health issues and practise preventative care (Woodward, Hutchinson, Abelson & Norman, 1996a). Women are less likely than men to work in rural areas, but when they do, they are more likely than men to attend births. They put in as many hours as their male counterparts and more than women in urban areas (Incitti, Rouke, Rouke & Kennard, 2003).

Thus, the way women tend to practise medicine may mean better care. That they tend to take more time is particularly important. According to interviewees in the Women and Health Care Reform project on how women define quality care (see Chapter 9), taking time to understand the whole person and her specific issues was their highest priority in quality care. In Atlantic Canada, a doctor was described as excellent because "she'll sit down with me for half an hour if I need to ask questions and depending on what I need." A young Caucasian graduate student likes her doctor "because when I go in, she sits down and looks at my chart and, you know, she asks me what I'm up to now and stuff like that. So she takes the time to work with me." Many women prefer to deal with a woman physician simply because she is a woman and this is especially the case for lesbian women (Geddes, 1994) and women from certain religious groups. The growing number of women in medicine therefore necessarily improves women's access to care, but the research on gender has focused more on the number of patients seen—defined in terms of productivity rather than in terms of the effect of women's approaches to care.

It is clear nevertheless that the pressures women face are often different than those of men. There is convincing research to demonstrate that under current conditions women physicians take more responsibility for children and domestic work than do male physicians, although men in general are doing more at home compared to what they once did (Woodward, Hutchinson, Abelson & Norman, 1996b; Woodward, Ferrier, Cohen & Brown, 2001). Moreover, male physicians seldom take time away from their paid work to care for their children. "The difference in work hours between men and women was lowest at age 25 to 29 and was the most noticeable at 35 to 44" (CIHI, 2007, 63); in other words, during the years of child care. As a result, women "put in many more hours in combining professional duties, childcare and household responsibilities" (Herbert, Whiteside, McKnight, Verma & Wilson, 2008, 659). According to a 2000 study (Cujec, Oancia, Bohm & Johnson, 2000), women in medical school, in residency programs, and in academic medical positions were less likely than men in similar positions to recommend to others in medicine that they become parents. Compared to men in medicine, women were also more likely to delay having children in order to get through the gruelling hours of residency and the initial stages of setting up a practice.

Furthermore, although women have entered medicine in large numbers, their presence does not necessarily mean that problems of discrimination and sexual harassment disappear. As another editorial in the *Canadian Medical Association Journal* put it, "It requires courage as well as mental and moral energy to deal effectively with sexual harassment, which, unfortunately, remains prevalent in medical schools as well as in academic medicine" (Palepu & Herbert, 2002, 8). A Canadian study found that a third of women physicians interviewed had been physically assaulted and over 70 percent had experienced verbal abuse. Nearly half said they faced unusually high levels of stress and 17 percent took antidepressant drugs. The women attributed these health issues both to their double day of work and to their work environments (Stewart, Ahmad, Cheung, Bergman & Dell, 2000). Some of this stress may be attributed to the continuing pressure of health care reforms and efforts to reduce doctors' power, but some of it is the result of gender relations at work. It is interesting to note that gender relations are also at play in terms of the nurse-doctor relationship. Nurses are less willing to defer to female physicians and, while this can mean more egalitarian encounters, it can also mean more hostility (Zelek & Phillips, 2003).

In addition, the fee structure has a gender impact. Women in medicine make less money than men not only because more women work part-time, but also because the fee structure rewards men's patterns of work. Specialists are paid more than doctors in primary care, where most women work, and male-dominated specialties are paid more than female-dominated ones. The fee-for-service structure is based both on how many patients are seen and their diagnosis. Women have lower incomes in part because they take more time with patients and because they spend more time on prevention and mental health, which pay less than many treatment-based services.

The distribution of physicians and surgeons also follows gender lines, and this segregation can have an impact on women seeking care. One example is orthopedic surgery. Even though women have greater need for such surgery, only 92 of the 1,235 orthopedic surgeons are women (CIHI, 2008, tables 2.1 and 2.2). Given evidence that male doctors are more likely to define men's than women's orthopedic problems as worthy of surgery (Jackson, Pederson & Boscoe, 2008), the lack of female specialists staffing the gates may help explain why many women do not get the surgery they need.

Solutions lie not in limiting the number of women practising medicine or in blaming women for limiting access. Rather, solutions must begin by recognizing that both male and female doctors need to care for their families and both need time in order to do so. The hours of work and the arrangements of shifts for doctors in both their education and practices can be changed, as Women's College Hospital in Toronto has shown with its flexible scheduling for doctors and its collaborative team approach (Daly et al., 2008). Solutions can also be found by providing more supports for women when they have children: supports such as daycare, flexible hours, and paid maternity leave. For example, Ontario women physicians negotiated parental leave benefits with the government in 2000 (Lent, Phillips, Richardson & Stewart, 2000), and residents in hospitals then became eligible for benefits under Employment Insurance. Equally important, we need to assess the impact on health of women's ways of practising medicine instead of assuming that, for example, the longer time they spend with patients is a problem.

In sum, the dramatic increase in the number of women that followed the removal of quotas on women in medical school has been a subject of interest and has led to conflicting conclusions. Although women may work fewer hours, see fewer patients than men, work in different specialties, and be less likely to practise in rural areas, the growing number of women doctors means more women have access to the services they need and more can see a female physician. The increasing number of women may also mean that women get a different kind of care, care that may well better suit their needs. For the women who practise medicine, gender constraints still often apply and add to the stress of their work.

# Nurses

The issues are somewhat different in the case of nurses. Nurses are generally not gatekeepers to the health care system. They are, however, the single largest occupational category in health services, with registered nurses (RNs) and licensed practical nurses (LPNs) accounting for 43 percent of all those included in Statistics Canada's definition of health personnel (CIHI, 2007, Figure 3.2). Nurses play a central role in the provision of daily care. Indeed, research has demonstrated that "when the number of working nurses falls, patient deaths and other adverse incidences increase.

Whether measured as nurse-to-patient ratios or hours worked per patient, fewer nurses are associated with poorer care" (Canadian Health Services Research Foundation [CHSRF], 2006, 1). As is the case with doctors, their numbers, their location, training, and conditions of work shape women's access to care. Given that more than nine out of 10 nurses are women, nursing is undoubtedly women's work. Indeed, the very fact of women's numerical dominance may account for the limited amount of explicit attention paid to gender in the health human resources literature on nursing. The virtual absence of men may also be a factor because much of the research on women is based on male-to-female comparisons.

Nineteenth-century efforts to make nursing a respectable job for women were based on the twin but somewhat contradictory assumptions that women were particularly suited for such work, and that they needed education to acquire the requisite skills for the job (Bates, Dodd & Rousseau, 2005). More recent efforts have focused on distancing nursing from an association with women's "innate" skills and even from an association with women's work. The newer emphasis on evidence-based nursing and on university education can be seen as attempts not only to enhance the effectiveness of nursing, but also to define nursing as a profession—like the male-dominated ones—based on science and formal training. Similarly, nursing organizations' continuing efforts to shed tasks such as cleaning and feeding, which have long been associated with women's work in the home, can be understood as a means of disassociating the work from women, as well as a means of making the job more attractive (Armstrong & Armstrong, 2009). The debates within nursing about whether or not nurses should emphasize caring as a central component that distinguishes their work from that of doctors have undertones of old debates about women's natural empathy. Yet nursing in Canada is still something women do. A recent article (Ryckewaert, 2010), titled "Nursing: Not Necessarily Women's Work," speaks volumes about current assumptions when it quotes a male student saying that men in nursing "aren't all gay, they aren't failed doctors, and they aren't doing 'women's work.' But they are a rare species in Canada." The association with women's work is understood to be an association with unskilled work of little market value.

Nurses have been more successful in using their collective strength to improve their pay, benefits, and conditions of work (Armstrong & Silas, 2010). Resisting the notion that nursing is a woman's labour of love that is its own reward, nurses began to organize into unions after the Second World War. Although a significant number of nurses objected to the move on the grounds of women's commitment to patients, others argued that nurses could provide appropriate patient care only if they had decent working conditions. Today, 80 percent of Canadian nurses are covered by union contracts, and many of those without unions benefit from union negotiations (Armstrong & Silas, 2010). Along with women in other jobs, nurses fought for and gained the right to stay in the job after marriage and pregnancy. They won seniority rights that allowed them to plan ahead and the right to resist unfair treatment from doctors and other employers. These victories help explain why most nurses are now over 40 (CIHI, 2010a, Table 9), the first time we have ever seen a nursing workforce made up primarily of older women.

This is not to suggest that unions have been completely successful in protecting nurses' jobs and conditions of work. Nurses have been leaving nursing in large numbers, primarily because of working conditions. Young nurses have been dropping out, both because the workload is too heavy and because current conditions mean they cannot practise the kind of nursing they had been taught as essential to good care. "Research showed that within the first five years of graduation, we were losing between two and three nurses for every five graduates" (Hamilton, 2007, 3). Older nurses are leaving for similar reasons, and age combined with the increasingly heavy workloads makes the work even harder for them.

Nurses are not only facing heavy demands during their regular hours of work. Official overtime increased by 20 percent between 2002 and 2004, creating particular problems for women who carry the bulk of their household's domestic responsibilities (Hamilton, 2007). Official data can hide even higher extra hours. Research by Donna Baines (2004) shows that official overtime hides the many extra hours of unpaid work done by women in their paid jobs. Women social workers are more likely than men to put in extra hours because they feel responsible for, and are held responsible for their patients. Similar patterns appear in nursing. Women nurses are more likely than male nurses to arrive early or stay late and to work through breaks (Statistics Canada, 2007). According to Statistics Canada survey data, 37 percent of female nurses usually work over 40 hours a week, and more than one in four worked shifts of 12 hours or more (Statistics Canada, 2007). The majority had no flexibility in the days or hours worked and did not even know a week ahead what their schedules would be (Statistics Canada, 2007).

This overwork shows up in women's health. Female nurses are much more likely than male nurses to suffer from migraines, cancer, and ulcers, for example (Statistics Canada, 2007). That they are also more likely to suffer from these conditions than other women suggests the problem is not biological. The increasing pressures from work speed-up and overtime make it particularly difficult for women nurses, given their other job at home. Women are leaving as a result.

It is not only working conditions that prompt women to leave nursing. Nurses also leave their jobs because of the racism they experience. Responses to an Ontario survey (Das Gupta, 2009) indicate that most nurses of colour experience "everyday forms of racism." The primary sources are "colleagues, followed by patients, doctors, managers and others" (p. 114). Those born outside Canada may face particular forms of discrimination. "In 2006, more than 20,000 licensed practical nurses and registered nurses working in Canada (not including Quebec) had graduated outside Canada" (Hoag, 2008, 271). The Philippines was the most important source, "followed by the United Kingdom, the United States, India and Hong Kong. The proportion of internationally educated registered nurses grew from 7% (15,659) in 2001 to 8% (19,230) in 2005" (Hoag, 2008, 271). But many with foreign credentials have significant difficulty having those credentials recognized in Canada, and the exams set by Canadian nurses' organizations are often a major barrier to entry (Stasiulis & Bakan, 2005, Chapter 6). Racism may also help explain why Aboriginal women are under-represented in health services (CIHI, 2007).

The issue of foreign trained nurses is complicated. Canadian nurses argue that in testing those who are foreign trained they are simply seeking to uphold standards. Canadian nurses may also resist the hiring of those who are foreign trained because nurses from other countries can be used to fill vacancies created in Canada as a result of working conditions. In other words, nurses may be hired from other countries instead of addressing the conditions that make women already in Canada leave nursing. This view is supported by the evidence on the number of nurses who do not work as nurses. More than 10,000 Canadian-educated nurses are not seeking employment in nursing (CIHI, 2010a, Table 3). This is often a result of working conditions, what they see as the under-valuing of this women's work, and the assumption that because they are women they can multi-task, taking on the jobs left by others (McIntyre & McDonald, 2010). Nurses' organizations also worry about the stripping of resources in other countries. Foreign-educated nurses often leave their own children at home to be cared for by other women at the same time as their home countries are left without adequate supplies of nurses.

Nurses' collective efforts have an impact on women's health and access to care. Unions have helped improve the quality of care through their efforts to protect women who are nurses. A US study demonstrates the value of these protections, showing a relationship between positive patient outcomes and unionization (Seago & Ash, 2002). The expansion of the nurse practitioner program is also an example of nurses working to protect their interests in ways that benefit women, given that nurse practitioners provide services used more by women than by men (Horrocks, Anderson & Salisbury, 2002). In addition, research has shown that nurse practitioners kept better records and communicated more effectively with patients than doctors while taking more time to provide advice on self-care and the management of chronic health conditions of the sort that plague women (Horrocks, Anderson & Salisbury, 2002). Like nurse practitioners, nurses in general are more likely to serve rural areas. Indeed, while doctors tend to be clustered in major urban areas, nurses are distributed among services and across the country in relative proportion to the population.

Nurses continue to struggle to provide good care and maintain access. However, nurses have not been able to resist many of the reforms that have made it harder for them to provide quality care. Patient stays have been shortened. Fewer nurses are expected to provide care for people with increasingly complicated care needs, often under surveillance from managers. Homecare nurses are left alone to deal with increasingly complex care provided in varying types of homes, some of them dangerous. As a result, more than one in 10 nurses surveyed by Statistics Canada (2007) reported their team delivered fair or poor care. Although there is growing evidence of the importance of the issues discussed above, the Statistics Canada survey did not ask about training in women's issues or in issues related to racism. Moreover, nurses' programs do not usually educate nurses in gender-based analysis or in an approach to women's health issues that goes beyond reproduction to understand all issues as women's issues. Attention is often dedicated to cultural competency, but not necessarily to the analysis of oppressions.

In sum, nursing remains women's work. Nurses have organized in ways that have improved their pay and working conditions and the result is better care for women. Problems not only remain, but have expanded with recent reforms that have increased workloads and intensified care work. There is still little gender-based analysis in nurses' education or in the organizations that represent them. Indeed, there have been attempts to dissociate nursing from women's work rather than confront the notion that work done

primarily by women is usually unskilled and biologically determined rather than learned.

## Other Health Services Workers

Nurses and doctors still make up the majority of those recognized as "health personnel" by CIHI and Statistics Canada. The
proportion of health care workers in "other health personnel"
categories, however, is steadily growing. At the same time, many
others working in health services are no longer counted as part
of the health care labour force. By 2005, technologists and technicians, social workers and therapists, along with dentists and their
assistants, chiropractors, midwives, pharmacists, and dieticians
accounted for 48 percent of health providers as defined by CIHI
(CIHI, 2007). These are most of the people that Statistics Canada
calls "other health personnel." Although the CIHI figures include
some health records administrators, the data leave out most other
clerical workers, as well as those who cook, clean, do laundry,
and provide much of the direct care as personnel support workers. Yet, as Women and Health Care Reform (2009) demonstrated
in our workshop and popular piece on the workers who are frequently termed "ancillary," food, clothing, and the physical environment are critical to everyone's health. Indeed, factors such as
cleaning and nutrition are even more important to those who are
particularly vulnerable as a result of illness, and the nature of
the work changes when it is done within health services. Record
keeping, too, takes on particular significance in care work. Most
of those who do this "ancillary" work are women and they are
now close to a majority of those employed in health and social
services (Armstrong, Armstrong & Scott Dixon, 2008). For these
reasons the final section of this chapter looks at all other health
care workers in order to explore the gender issues for both those
who provide and those who receive care.

Those classified as in "other occupations in health" or "other health personnel" by Statistics Canada and CIHI are segregated by sex in terms of both jobs and workplaces (CIHI, 2007). According to CIHI (2007) data, more than 90 percent of dental assistants, hygienists, and therapists are women, and this is also the case for dieticians and nutritionists, speech pathologists, and occupational therapists. Eighty percent or more of the clerks, sonographers, laboratory and other technicians are women, and so are nearly four out of five social workers and physiotherapists. Meanwhile, men are the majority of chiropractors, dentists, other administrative service managers, and optometrists.

What is important to note about this division of labour is that the female-dominated occupations are, for the most part, ones that are directed, managed, or supervised by the male-dominated ones. Power is not equally shared in health services despite the large number of women. Although women account for over 80 percent of all those employed in health care, they make up just 51 percent of senior managers. As managers, women are heavily concentrated in smaller establishments and in long-term care, where the work involves fewer employees and brings less prestige, authority, and remuneration. Moreover, many of these "other occupations in health" involve spending significant time with those needing care as is the case with nurses, but with someone else in charge. Dental hygienists, for example, often spend an hour cleaning teeth and taking X-rays, followed by a short check by the dentists.

While this pattern of segregation has changed little over the years, there are some exceptions. Women have moved into pharmacy, where they have quickly become a majority (CIHI, 2009a). This movement has happened at the same time as the work has been transformed from one in which most pharmacists own the store to one in which the majority are employees. In other words, women have moved into this profession just as the profession itself lost some power and prestige. At the same time, however, working as an employee may allow women more control over their time and thus make it easier to accommodate the demands of their families. Equally important, as pharmacists focus more on providing advice, women may feel more comfortable being served by another woman. Plan B, known as the morning-after pill, can now be dispensed by pharmacists, providing an obvious example of a case where service from a woman might be preferred.

Another major change in the division of labour has been the expansion of midwifery (see Chapter 4 for a broader discussion of maternity care). A report from CIHI (2009a) estimates that in 2008, there were approximately 600 registered midwives and all of them were women. This represents a significant increase from the 370 counted in 2001 (CIHI, 2009a) and clearly has important implications for women's access to care. As is the case with nurse practitioners, midwives in Canada are still struggling to establish their place in relation to doctors and nurses, however, and are not always supported by these colleagues or funded appropriately by the government.

Like nurses, women in these other professional occupations have been organizing to defend their rights. And like nurses, they have often had internal debates about the models to follow and the extent to which they should form professional associations or unions and distance themselves from gender issues. Some have sought to make registration compulsory while others have resisted; some have been regulated by provinces and worked for such regulation while others have been opposed. Supporters of regulation and registration argue that it will ensure quality. Opponents often describe the regulated professions as monopolies that inappropriately limit entry, copying male models of practice and requiring lengthy training processes that make it difficult for many women to join. Just as the movement of nursing education out of hospitals and into post-secondary educational institutions meant poor women found it harder to become nurses, so too can the requirement for more formal training restrict access to the emerging occupations for women without financial means or whose families oppose such education for women.

The jobs included by Statistics Canada in the "other health personnel" category are all ones that require formal training, whether or not they are regulated or require registration. This classification suggests that skills are only required and should only be recognized if they are learned and accredited in an academic setting. The credentials help establish at least some of the work as skilled. This contrasts with the jobs increasingly defined as ancillary (Armstrong, Armstrong & Scott-Dixon, 2008). Those who cook, clean, do laundry, and provide personal care in health services seldom have formal training recognized or formally required in their jobs. They do work long defined as unskilled.

In the past, those who cook, clean, do laundry, keep records, and those providing direct personal care were at least included in the Statistics Canada industry data, which were based on where people worked as opposed to what they do at work (captured by the occupational data). Increasingly, industry is defined by the employer rather than the workplace, so many of these workers disappear from health services because their jobs have been contracted out to private employers. This is not just an esoteric counting issue of concern only to statisticians. It reflects strategies based on defining this work out of care and reclassifying these jobs as hotel work so it can be contracted out to private companies in the hospitality sector at lower cost. Yet defining some health sector workers out of care work ignores their critical contribution to the success of interventions, to recovery, and to sustaining health and preventing illness or disability. This lack of attention has negative consequences for health and care. Marjorie Cohen (2001) has convincingly demonstrated that ancillary health care workers cannot be defined or treated as hospitality workers, both because health care requires different skills and because such workers form an integral part of health care teams. Others have shown how the failure to recognize the importance of the work and the skills involved often means contracting out that leads not only to significant health problems, but to higher costs (Davies, 2005). The experience with SARS demonstrated that cleanliness is critical to care and requires particular kinds of skills within health services, although not all health services have applied this lesson.

These approaches to and definitions of ancillary work reflect assumptions about gender, especially about skills and women's work. It is work associated with the home and traditionally done by women, although it is sometimes done by marginalized men. The women who do the work seldom have formal credentials directly related to the work or formal training for the job. In Canada, however, most have completed high school and a significant number have further education, education that may help them do the work well. Most have had training in the job and a majority have gained skills through experience as well (Armstrong, Armstrong & Scott-Dixon, 2008). Associated as it is with women's work in the home, the skills, effort, responsibilities, and working conditions involved remain invisible and undervalued. This invisibility and undervaluing contributes to the process of defining ancillary work out of care work. Women's lack of power contributes to this process, and this is especially the case for the most marginalized women. Many of the women who do this work are recent immigrants and/or are racialized.

It would be a mistake to assume that the women who do this ancillary work have simply accepted their fate. Those in hospitals have unionized and struggled hard to improve their conditions of work and the recognition of their skills. As a result, women who do ancillary work in health services have better pay, security, and benefits than those doing similarly classified work in the private sector (Armstrong & Laxer, 2006). Contracting out has undermined some of these gains and the increasing numbers of those who work in home care are hard to organize because they do not work together in one workplace (Denton et al., 2006). Nevertheless, the women who do this work may gain some power as a result of the growing demand for providers, especially in personal care, and of union efforts to protect their rights.

In short, those in "other health care services" constitute the majority of those working in care, they are overwhelmingly women, and they are often counted out of care work. Their invisibility needs to be understood in terms of women's work and lack of power.

# The Unpaid Labour Force

The contribution of the vast army of unpaid caregivers is even less visible than that of ancillary health care workers. Indeed, more care work is unpaid than paid. Estimates vary because the work is often hidden in the household, but it is clear that the presence of paid care workers does not mean that unpaid care is absent. According to CIHI (2010b), 98 percent of seniors receiving care paid for from the public purse also had one or more unpaid care providers. Recent estimates indicate that the cost of replacing those who provide unpaid care for the elderly with those hired to assist with activities of daily living would amount to $25 billion a year (Hollander, Liu & Chappell, 2009). And these figures do not include the many who care for children with disabilities or who work as volunteers in health care facilities. This army of unpaid caregivers is made up primarily of women, although data on unpaid work collected since 1996 indicate men have been doing more unpaid care (Grant et al., 2004). Although Chapter 5 on long-term care and Chapter 6 on home care also take up the issue of unpaid care work, it is essential to include a discussion here not only because such work accounts for the majority of care, but also because it influences and is influenced by paid care work.

The data on unpaid care provision need to be examined carefully to see the patterns by gender. A 2010 study of Canadians aged 45 and over shows that "While equal proportions of men and women were caregivers, women were more likely to be primary caregivers (31%) than were men (20%)" (Lilly, Laporte & Coyte, 2010, 4). When men were primary caregivers, they provided fewer hours of care, an average of 11 hours a week compared to 16 for women (Lilly, Laporte & Coyte, 2010). Unlike the men who were primary caregivers, women said there were no substitutes available to do the work when they took on the primary responsibility. As Aronson (1992) makes clear, this lack of substitutes builds on and reinforces women's sense of responsibility for care.

Women not only provide more unpaid care than men, but also do different kinds of unpaid care. For example, a 2004 survey found that 70 percent of those providing unpaid care for someone with a mental illness were women, and the proportion of women who look after more than one person when they do so is almost twice that of men (Decima, 2004). Women were also significantly more likely than men to look after parents with mental health problems. Men mainly provide care for partners, although women's greater longevity and tendency to marry men older than themselves mean there are more women than men looking after spouses. A third of the women, compared to a quarter of the men, looked after someone with schizophrenia, while men were more likely to deal with mood disorders. A large majority of both women and men felt that providing care for those with mental health problems is a family responsibility, although of men, "(28%) are more likely than women (17%) to feel that other options were available to them when they decided to be the primary caregiver" (Decima, 2004, 5). In other words, women do more and heavier care, but have less choice about providing that care.

A study of employed people who also provided unpaid care reveals both important differences among women and the consequences of such a double load for women (Duxbury, Higgins & Shroeder, 2009). According to this research, money matters a lot. Those particularly subject to physical strain were older women who lived with those for whom they provided care and who were unable to pay for support or quit their paid work. Emotional strain was highest for women with little money, without children, and providing care for elderly dependants. With the work characterized as high demand and low control over the job, it is not surprising that women's health, as well as their paid work, suffers when they provide unpaid care. Unfortunately, this study did not look at the intersection of gender and other social locations.

One way strain plays out is in conflict with the other women who provide some paid care. It plays out in home care in part because the situation can invite conflict over skills and definitions of appropriate care. Those paid to do the work often have years of formal training and may resent being asked to teach others in minutes what these professionals have taken years to learn. Meanwhile, the women who provide unpaid care may resent the failure to recognize the skills they have learned and their knowledge of the person needing care. As McKeever (1999) explains,

> [the] chain of relationships links government and corporate interests to paid health-care workers, unpaid family caregivers, and people who have long-term care needs. At the bottom are family caregivers whose work has been appropriated from the domestic sphere and substituted for formerly paid nursing work. (p. 185)

Equally important, strains often result from the ways people from racialized groups are treated as unpaid providers of care.

Another way strain may become visible is in poor care or even abuse of the women who need care. Elderly women and women with disabilities are particularly vulnerable to abuse or neglect, given that they are often physically and economically dependent on those who provide unpaid care (Driedger & Owen, 2008). As chapters 5 and 6 make clear, for too many women there is not enough care.

In sum, unpaid workers make up the bulk of the health care labour force. Most of the women who bear primary responsibility for care are women who have few options in terms of providing care, and the work often takes a heavy toll on their health. Care work, paid or unpaid, can be rewarding, but it requires supports and an element of choice. *The Charlottetown Declaration on the Right to Care* (Appendix 1) is intended to set out the principles on which care should be based so that women do not suffer as unpaid providers, and those who need the care do not suffer either.

# Conclusions

Gender plays a central role in who works in care, who counts as health care workers, the care to which women have access, and the care they receive. More doctors are women than in the past, with complex and often positive consequences for care. Almost all nurses are women, and this too can mean positive consequences. The nursing workforce is aging, in large measure because this is the generation that successfully demanded the right to stay in paid work even after marriage and pregnancy. As a large but shrinking proportion of the health care labour force, nurses increasingly face conditions that leave them making up for the care deficit and working harder even as age and unpaid care responsibilities may make the pressures more difficult to handle. Those defined as "other health care personnel" by Statistics Canada and CIHI mainly work under the instructions of those defined as professional, doing the kind of assisting work long assigned to women. But the largest proportion of the paid workforce is being defined out of care work, and is dismissed as doing unskilled women's work. A growing number of these workers provide the hands-on care as personal care providers. At the same time, women without formal training provide the major share of unpaid care, work that is expanding as more and more complex care is sent home. As a result of the changing conditions and locations of work described here and in other chapters throughout the book, those with care needs may be put at risk along with those who provide care. Without gender analysis, it is difficult to understand the developments in care and care work. We have enough data to know that gender matters, but we need to know more about how gender is at play, and about the differences among women working in care.

# References

Armstrong, P. (1993). Professions, unions, or what? Learning from nurses. In L. Briskin & P. McDermott (Eds.), *Women challenging unions* (pp. 304–324). Toronto: University of Toronto Press.

Armstrong, P. & Armstrong, H. (2009). Contradictions at work: Struggles for control in Canadian health care. In L. Panitch & C. Leys (Eds.), *Morbid symptoms: Health under capitalism: Socialist Register 2010* (pp. 145–167). London: Monthly Review Press.

Armstrong, P., Armstrong, H. & Scott-Dixon, K. (2008). *Critical to care: The invisible women in health services.* Toronto: University of Toronto Press.

Armstrong, P. & Laxer, K. (2006) Precarious work, privatization, and the health care industry: The case of ancillary workers. In L. Vosko (Ed.), *Precarious employment: Understanding labour market insecurity in Canada* (pp. 115–138). Montreal: McGill-Queen's University Press.

Armstrong, P. & Silas, L. (2010). Taking power: Making change. Nurses' unions in Canada. In M. McIntyre & C. McDonald (Eds.), *Realities of Canadian nursing: Professional, practice, and power issues* (pp. 316–336). New York: Lippincott Williams & Wilkins.

Aronson, J. (1992). Women's sense of responsibility for the care of old people. "But who else is going to do it?" *Gender and Society 6*(1), 8–22.

Baines, D. (2004). Caring for nothing: Work organization and unwaged labour in social services. *Work, Employment, and Society 18*(2), 267–295.

Bates, C., Dodd, D. & Rosseau, N. (Eds.). (2005). *On all frontiers: Four centuries of Canadian nursing.* Ottawa: University of Ottawa Press.

Blackwell, T. (2009, May 19). *Female doctors hurt productivity: Report. National Post.* Retrieved from http://www.nationalpost.com/news/story

Canadian Health Services Research Foundation (CHSRF). (2006). *Implement nurse staffing plans for better quality of care. Evidence boost.* Retrieved from *http://www.chsrf.ca/mythbusters/html/boost7_e.php-*

Canadian Institute for Health Information (CIHI). (2007). *Canada's health care providers, 2007*. Ottawa: CIHI.

Canadian Institute for Health Information (CIHI). (2008). *Supply distribution and migration of Canadian physicians, 2007*. Ottawa: CIHI.

Canadian Institute for Health Information (CIHI). (2009a). *Canada's health care providers — 2008 provincial profiles: A look at 24 health occupations*. Ottawa: CIHI.

Canadian Institute for Health Information (CIHI). (2009b). *Supply, distribution, and migration of Canadian physicians, 2008*. Ottawa: CIHI.

Canadian Institute for Health Information (CIHI). (2010a). *Regulated nurses: Canadian trends, 2004–2008. Updated February 2010*. Retrieved from http://secure.cihi.ca/cihiweb/products/regulated_nurses_2004_2008_en.pdf

Canadian Institute for Health Information (CIHI). (2010b). *Supporting informal caregivers — the heart of the home*. Ottawa: CIHI.

Cohen, M.G. (2001, October). *Do comparisons between hospital support workers and hospitality workers make sense?* Retrieved from http://www.heu.org/~DOCUMENTS/research_reports/ Comparison_Hospital_Support_Workers_1.pdf

Cujec, B., Oancia, T., Bohm, C. & Johnson, D. (2000). Career and parenting satisfaction among medical students, residents, and physician teachers at a Canadian medical school. *Canadian Medical Association Journal 162*(5), 637–640.

Daly, T., Armstrong, P., Armstrong, H., Braedley, S. & Oliver, V. (2008). *Contradictions: Health equity and women's health services in Toronto*. Toronto: Wellesley Institute.

Das Gupta, T. (2009). *Real nurses and others: Racism in nursing*. Halifax: Fernwood Publishing.

Davies, S. (2005). *Hospital contract cleaning and infection control*. Cardiff: School of Social Sciences, Cardiff University.

Decima. (2004). *Informal/ family caregivers in Canada caring for someone with a mental illness*. Retrieved from http://www.hc-sc.gc.ca/hcs-sss/pubs/home-domicile/2004-mental-care-soins/index-eng.php

Denton, M., Zeytinoglu, I., Davies, S. & Hunter, D. 2006. Where have all the homecare workers gone? In C. Beach, R. Chaykowski, S. Shortt, F. St-Hilaire & A. Sweetman (Eds.), *Health services restructuring in*

*Canada: New evidence and new directions* (pp. 245–268). Kingston: John Deutsch Institute, Queen's University and Montreal: Institute for Research on Public Policy.

Driedger, D. & Owen, M. (2008). *Dissonant disabilities: Women with chronic illnesses explore their lives.* Toronto: CPSI.

Duxbury, L., Higgins, C. & Shroeder, B. (2009). *Balancing paid work and caregiver responsibilities: A closer look at family caregivers in Canada.* Retrieved from http://www.cprn.org/documents/51061_EN.pdf

Geddes, V.A. (1994). Lesbian expectations and experiences with family doctors. How much does the physicians' sex matter? *Canadian Family Physician 40,* 908–920.

Grant, K.R., Amaratunga, C., Armstrong, P., Boscoe, M., Pederson, A. & Willson, K. (Eds.). (2004). *Caring for/caring about: Women, homecare, and unpaid caregiving.* Aurora: Garamond.

Gulli, C. & Lunau, K. (2008, January 2). Adding fuel to the doctor crisis. *Maclean's 17,* 23–34.

Hamilton, N. (2007, February). Working conditions: An underlying policy issue. *Health Policy Research Bulletin 13,* 3–6.

Herbert, C., Whiteside, C., McKnight, D., Verma, S. & Wilson, L. (2008). Ending the sexist blame game. *Canadian Medical Association Journal 178*(6), 659.

Hoag, H. (2008). Canada increasingly reliant on foreign-trained health professionals. *Canadian Medical Association Journal 178*(3), 270–271.

Hollander, M.J., Liu, G. & Chappell, N.L. (2009). Who cares and how much? The imputed economic contribution to the Canadian healthcare system of middle-aged and older unpaid caregivers providing care for the elderly. *Healthcare Quarterly 12*(2), 42–49.

Horrocks, S., Anderson, C. & Salisbury, C. (2002). Systematic review of whether nurse practitioners working in primary care can provide equivalent care to doctors. *British Medical Journal 324,* 819–823.

Incitti, F., Rouke, J., Rouke, L.L. & Kennard, M. (2003). Rural women family physicians: Are they unique? *Canadian Family Physician 49*(3), 320–327.

Jackson, B., Pederson, A. & Boscoe, M. (2008). Waiting to wait: Improving wait times evidence through gender-based analysis. In P. Armstrong & J. Deadman (Eds.), *Women's health: Intersections of policy, research, and practice* (pp. 35–52). Toronto: Women's Press.

Lent, B., Phillips, S.P., Richardson, B. & Stewart, D. (2000). Promoting parental leave for female and male physicians. *Canadian Medical Association Journal 162*(11), 1575–1576.

Lilly, M.B., Laporte, A. & Coyte, P.C. (2010). Do they care too much to work? The influence of caregiving intensity on the labour force participation of unpaid caregivers. *Canadian Journal of Health Economics 29*(6), 895–903.

Maheux, B., Haley, N., Rivard, M. & Gervais, A. (1997). Do women physicians do more STD prevention than men? Quebec study of recently trained family physicians. *Canadian Family Physician 43*, 1089–1095.

McIntyre, M. & McDonald, C. (2010). The nursing shortage: Assumptions and realities. In M. McIntyre & C. McDonald (Eds.), *Realities of Canadian nursing: Professional, practice, and power issues* (pp. 303–315). NewYork: Lippincott Williams & Wilkins.

McKeever, P. (1999). Between women: Nurses and family caregivers. *Canadian Journal of Nursing Research 30*(4), 185–191.

Palepu, A. & Herbert, C.P. (2002). Medical women in academia: The silences we keep. *Canadian Medical Association Journal 167*(8), 877–879.

Roter, D.L., Hall, J.A. & Aoki, Y. (2002). Physician gender effects in medical communications. *JAMA: The Journal of the American Medical Association 288*(6), 756–764.

Ryckewaert, L. (2010, April 6). Nursing work: Not necessarily women's work. *University Affairs*. Retrieved from http://ww.universityaffairs.ca/nursing-not-necessarily-women's work.aspx

Seago, J.A. & Ash, M. (2002). Registered nurse union and patient outcomes. *Journal of Nursing Administration 32*(3), 143–151.

Stasiulis, D. & Bakan, A. (2005). *Negotiating citizenship: Migrant women in Canada and the global system*. Toronto: University of Toronto Press.

Statistics Canada. (2007). *2005 National Survey of the Work and Health of Nurses*. Ottawa: Health Canada.

Stewart, D.E., Ahmad, F., Cheung, A.M., Bergman, B. & Dell, D.L. (2000). Women physicians and stress. *Journal of Women's Health and Gender-Based Medicine 9*(2), 185–190.

Weizblit, N., Noble, J. & Baerlocher, M. (2009). The feminization of medicine and its impact upon doctor productivity. *Medical Education* 43(5), 442–448.

Women and Health Care Reform. (2009). *Ancillary health care work.* Retrieved from http://www.womenandhealthcarereform.ca/en/work_ancillary.html

Woodward, C.A., Ferrier, B., Cohen, M. & Brown, J. (2001). Professional activity: How is family physicians' work time changing? *Canadian Family Physician 47*, 1414–1421.

Woodward, C.A., Hutchison, B.G., Abelson, J. & Norman, G. (1996a). Do female primary care physicians practise preventive care differently from their male colleagues? *Canadian Family Physician 42*, 2370–2379.

Woodward, C.A., Hutchinson, B.G., Abelson, J. & Norman, G. (1996b). Time spent on professional activities and unwaged domestic work: Is it different for male and female primary care physicians who have children at home? *Canadian Family Physician 42*, 1928–1935.

Zelek, B. & Phillips, S.P. (2003). Gender and power: Nurses and doctors in Canada. *International Journal for Equity in Health 2*(1). Retrieved from http://www.ncbi.nlm.nih.gov/pmc/articles/PMC150379/?log$=activity

Zukewich, N. (2003, Fall). Unpaid informal caregiving. *Canadian Social Trends 70*, 14–18.

## CHAPTER 8

# The Mental Health of Women Health Care Workers

PAT ARMSTRONG

The purpose of this book is to demonstrate the importance of a gender-based analysis, in part through taking up issues not usually examined from this perspective. The mental health of health care workers is such an issue. While women's mental health has received considerable attention, the mental health of health care workers has been less a matter of concern. When the mental health of health care workers is a focus of research, it has seldom been analyzed from a gender perspective. Issues of mental health arise in many of the chapters in this book, but starting with mental health issues allows us to see how a gender lens can expose critical aspects of work in care at the same time as it helps us understand why they have received so little attention.

Speaking as the chair of the Mental Health Commission of Canada, Dr. Michael Kirby (2008) identified the mental health of health care workers as a critical issue. He was referring specifically to "mental health care providers," but the argument holds for all those who provide care and who work in care. Indeed, on the basis of their research with health care workers (HCW) in British Columbia, Annalee Yassi and Tina Hancock (2005) conclude that "Mental disorders are the fastest growing cause of long-term disability in HCWs in BC, as elsewhere" (p. 35). It is important to note that only the severest cases result in long-term disability, hiding the many cases of workers who suffer in silence. Equally important, Yassi and Hancock's research focused exclusively on those paid to provide care. The large number who do unpaid care work are missing from the picture and excluded from long-term disability compensation.

Although there is a growing body of research demonstrating that mental health issues are not only common but growing among those who provide care, very little of this research takes gender into account. Most research on occupational health and safety, including the impact on mental health, has been "one-eyed," as Karen Messing (1998) puts it, focusing on the occupational health hazards men face and on the workplaces where men work. When we do have research on female-dominated workplaces, it does not often look at gender. Part of the problem may be the idea that gender research necessarily involves a comparison between women and men. Given that there are so few men involved in direct care work, comparative research is limited. The very fact that women are the overwhelming majority of care providers may help explain why little research on occupational health focuses on gender, especially when combined with the assumption that mental health problems are primarily the result of women's minds and bodies (Nasser, Baistow & Treasure, 2007). Part of the problem relates to the fact that the impact of care work on health does not tend to be immediate and visible, especially in the case of mental health. The mental health hazards for women are rendered invisible, too, by the cumulative nature of the impact, with health problems emerging slowly over time. This invisibility contrasts with the visibility of sudden death or obvious physical injuries that are more common in male-dominated work.

The purpose of this chapter is to show that gender must be central to our understanding of mental health issues, rather than to provide a definitive analysis of these issues in all their complexity. It takes up the questions raised in other chapters by asking: Why is this a woman's issue, what are the issues for women, and which women in what circumstances are affected? It concludes by raising questions that we need to address in order to improve the mental health of women health care workers. The chapter draws not only on the literature and some primary research but also on presentations given at a 1998 Vancouver workshop on mental health issues for women health care workers organized by Women and Health Care Reform in partnership with the BC Centre of Excellence for Women's Health. Although workshop participants had expertise in mental health and in gender-based analysis, we were surprised by how hard it was to maintain a focus that combined the issues of mental health, health care work, and gender. The difficulty reflects the divisions within the research, which tends to treat all these issues separately rather than in combination.

For the purposes of this chapter, mental health issues are broadly defined to include anxiety, depression, undue stress, and addictions, as well as other more traditional diagnoses. But mental health is not only about illness. Quoting the Minister of Public Works and Government Services Canada, Madeleine Dion Stout (2008), a member of the Mental Health Commission, reminded us at the workshop that mental health should be more positively defined to include "a sense of emotional and spiritual well-being that respects the importance of culture, equity, social justice, interconnections and personal dignity" (p. 6). We also define health care workers broadly to include everyone who works in the health and social service sector, including those who cook, clean, do laundry and clerical work for pay, and those who provide unpaid care at home and in the community. Such an approach is in keeping with the literature on the determinants of health, which shows the critical roles that food, clean environments, records, and social supports play within care (Armstrong, Armstrong & Scott-Dixon, 2008).

A feminist political economy approach prompts us to connect personal issues of mental health with the relations and organizations of work, and to locate these relations and methods of organizing within the larger context of health care policy and pressures at the global, national, and local levels. It leads us to ask whose interests are served and to recognize that work relations are characterized by inequities that can be altered. The feminist part means understanding that paid and unpaid work both matter and are integrally related as well as gendered. It also means asking what role biology plays and how biology itself is shaped by both social relations and conditions (Fausto-Sterling, 2005, 2006). For strategic and analytical reasons, such an approach sometimes means talking about women as a group, while always asking which women are affected, and sometimes talking about particular groups of women.

## The Mental Health of Health Care Workers

Most of us spend the majority of our day doing work, so it is not surprising that workplaces shape our possibilities for good mental health. As the Scientific Advisory Committee to the Global Business and Economic Roundtable on Addiction and Mental Health (2002) put it, "The workplace as a social environment has a major influence on the mental health of all who labour within it. The same environment can also influence the likelihood that certain employees will develop addiction-related problems" (p. iii). In other words, the conditions and relations of work shape our mental health. But our paid workplaces are not the only factor influencing our mental health. As this report goes on to say, "At the same time, people bring personal problems to the workplace with them. These problems interact with different types of social environments in the workplace so that they are either more or less likely to result in threats to health and productivity" (p. iii). An emphasis on conditions and relations is not to suggest that other factors, such as genetic makeup and chemical responses, do not play a role, but rather that we need to look at our various workplaces and their interactions to understand mental health. We also need to think about women's unpaid work in the household and the impact on their paid jobs.

The roundtable report talks about work in general, but some recent research draws our attention to the specific case of health care work. One reason for this attention is that the health care sector is a major employer throughout the world. In Canada, more than one in 10 people counted as employed works in the health and social assistance sector (Statistics Canada, 2010). Another reason is that mental health problems are rising significantly among health care workers, reflected in the figures on long-term disability (Yassi & Hancock, 2005). Health and social care is now the sector with the highest number of days lost per worker per year due to illness or disability (CANSIM, 2009).[1] Of course, not all these absences can be attributed to mental health issues, although we do know that mental health problems often become physical health ones too. A 2006 Statistics Canada survey of nurses (Shields & Wilkins, 2006) found that one in 10 nurses had taken time off work for mental health reasons. Although only 6 percent of the nurses said they have fair to poor mental health, 9 percent said they used antidepressants. It is hard not to see the need for such drugs as an indicator of mental health problems. Registered practical nurses had higher rates than registered nurses, with 9 percent saying they had fair to poor mental health. These rates are higher than in the overall labour force, suggesting that health care work is a factor in nurses' poor mental health. Moreover, these numbers on poor mental health may tell only part of the story. Given that the Statistics Canada survey found "close to one-fifth of nurses reported that their mental health had made their workload difficult to handle during the previous month" (Shields & Wilkins, 2006, 64), there is every reason to believe a large number of nurses suffer mental health consequences from their work. The other missing part of the story is the rest of the health care labour force, which has not been subject to the same kind of detailed investigation. We do know, however, that the absences due to illness and disability are even higher among other women working in other services, and mental health is likely to be a factor in many cases (Statistics Canada, 2009, Table 3.3).

The impact of the rise in mental health issues is felt far beyond the individual health care worker. There are consequences for the women's families and friends, for the people for whom they provide care, and for the health system as a whole. Women take their problems home from work, and the problems make it difficult for women to do their work at home, as well as in the health care system. The costs to the system as a whole may be even less obvious, but nonetheless real. At the closing session of the workshop organized by Women and Health Care Reform, Larry Myette, former medical director at the Health Care Benefits Trust in British Columbia, reported that workplace health problems account for $1 billion of the $6 billion health care budget, and much of this expenditure is the result of or related to mental health issues.

But it is not only those paid to provide care who risk their own mental health. Feminist political economists have emphasized the importance of unpaid care and its centrality to understanding care work. Various studies have shown that between 85 percent and 90 percent of what is often termed "informal care" is provided outside the formal system (Denton, 1997). It is also important to note that these figures do not include the unpaid care that the paid care workers put in as unpaid overtime. Women care workers, more often than men, work through lunch and breaks, and stay long after their paid job is done (Baines, 2006). A growing body of research suggests that the impact on mental health of providing such care can be profound.

"Caregiving is associated with higher rates of most psychiatric disorders," according to a 1997 comparative study of those providing and those not providing unpaid care in Ontario (Cochrane, Goering & Rogers, 1997, 2005). This study found that these unpaid providers use the health care system for mental health problems twice as much as those not providing unpaid care. A 2002 study by the Public Health Agency of Canada found that eight in 10 family caregivers suffered from stress, with almost 30 percent describing this stress as significant. In their review of the literature on caregiver mental health, MacNeil et al. (2010) point out that the mental health consequences can vary with the nature of the problems faced by those needing care. Those dealing with family members with dementia, for example, are particularly vulnerable, with one in four care providers exhibiting symptoms that fit with a clinical diagnosis of anxiety. The consequences can also vary with the social location of providers and the supports they have in providing care. Care providers whose first language is neither English nor French are especially at risk (Meshefedjian, McCusker, Bellavance & Baumgarten, 1998). A Queen's University thesis suggests that immigrants may be particularly vulnerable to depression when they provide unpaid care, with those without outside help being especially vulnerable (Dhawan, 1998).

In sum, mental health has been identified as a growing and expensive issue in health care work, where women account for the overwhelming majority of the labour force. However, the annotated bibliography prepared as background for this chapter (Campbell, 2010) indicates that the Canadian research remains limited and tends to focus on those providing care to people who themselves suffer from mental health issues. We still need to figure out not only the size and shape of the mental health problems the whole range of health care workers face, but also to what extent these problems primarily reflect necessary demands in care and to what extent they reflect either the way work is organized or/and the assumptions made in providing care. Equally important, very little of this literature makes gender central to the analysis even though, as the next section seeks to make clear, gender plays a critical role.

# The Mental Health of Women Health Care Workers

There are several reasons why this growing problem should be viewed as a woman's issue. One has to do with who does the work while another has to do with how they do the work. A third reason relates to assumptions made about women and their often triple shifts as paid care workers, mothers, and unpaid providers. The final reason relates to women's physical makeup.

A fifth of all employed women work in the health and social service sector and, as the previous chapter explains, women account for over 80 percent of the health care labour force (Statistics Canada, 2010). More than nine out of 10 registered nurses and registered nursing assistants are women, and this is the case for therapists too (Canadian Institute for Health Information [CIHI], 2008, Appendix F). Women will soon be the majority of physicians, and they are currently almost all the personal care assistants. Women are also most of the cooks, cleaners, and dietary and laundry workers in health services (Armstrong, Armstrong & Scott-Dixon, 2008).

At the same time, women do the overwhelming majority of unpaid, personal care. While men are doing more unpaid care, especially when it comes to things like taking their mothers grocery shopping or caring for their male partner, women provide most of the care that is required every day and that involves feeding, changing, toileting, and bathing (Cranswick & Dosman, 2008). It is this kind of daily demand that is most likely to lead to mental health issues, especially if the women are isolated or lack material and social supports and services. Such isolation is particularly evident in the North and in rural areas, but can happen in urban areas as well, especially if women are immigrants.

As Cyndi Brannen, a research associate at Dalhousie University, put it in her presentation at the workshop, "If we had a superhero, she would be a caregiver." She went on to explain that the skills and effort involved in being a health care superhero remain hidden, and the stress and trauma are endured in silence, in large measure because this is women's work. In her study of women unpaid care providers for the Atlantic Centre of Excellence for Women's Health, Brannen (2006) found that "across caregiving types, ethnic groups and geographic location, many women reported that caregiving led to feelings of depression and helplessness" (p. 1). Indeed, research suggests that the problem is greater for women not only because they are more likely to provide the daily personal care required, but also because they have learned to be more empathetic in ways that can threaten their health. Just as important are the assumptions made about both how women provide care and how they should provide care. It is too often assumed that women will make up for care deficits and will do so in ways that put others first.

This experience of mental strain is partly about the work women do in care. Their experiences in and out of the labour force play an important part, and so do cultural meanings attached to women and their work. According to the European Agency's study *Gender Issues in Health and Safety at Work* (European Union [EU], 2003), women report more work-related stress: "Women are more exposed to some specific stressors because of: the type of work they do; their position in the hierarchy of work organizations; discrimination; sexual harassment; their situation outside work" (p. 47). This report also highlights the mental impact of bullying and violence, things women are much more likely than men to experience in their paid and unpaid care work.

Health care work could be the model for what the European Agency report is talking about. It is not viewed as dangerous or particularly stressful work, even though it has the highest rates of absence due to injury and illness, partly because it is women who do the work. Yet research shows that health care work is often accompanied by violence, discrimination, sexual assault, and workers' lack of control over planning their day exacerbates these stresses. Women are underrepresented in the decision-making positions, and struggle to do their other care work at home (Armstrong, Armstrong & Scott-Dixon, 2008; Armstrong et al., 2009). Moreover, conditions are deteriorating. Research from British Columbia shows that the increasingly heavy workloads accompanying health care reforms have a particularly negative impact on mental health (Koehoorn, Ibrahim, Hertzman, Ostry & Brown, 2009).

Violence is itself a risk to mental health, and there can be little doubt that those providing care face violence on a daily basis. More than a quarter of the nurses in the Statistics Canada survey reported they had been physically assaulted in the previous year

(Shields & Wilkins, 2006, Chart 3.5), and four out of 10 providing direct care said they had faced emotional abuse from a patient (Appendix, Table 22). Interestingly, male nurses were more likely than female nurses to report such abuse. Given that this pattern is contrary to research on violence, the data suggest that men are more likely to perceive actions as abusive while women are more likely to accept it as part of the job or as something they caused.

In our comparative study of direct care workers in long-term care, nearly half reported that physical violence occurred more or less every day, although they felt they had no time to or even the option to report it. Another quarter said that they experienced violence on a weekly basis (Armstrong et al., 2009). Writing in on a survey that was part of this study, one personal support worker described violence as "a day-to-day thing ... an everyday occurrence." According to our focus groups in that study, direct care workers seldom report the violence because they may be blamed, because they often blame themselves, because they are told to "suck it up" or "lighten up," the same reasons given by many women who face domestic violence. Like many of the conditions women face at work, violence is often understood by managers and the women themselves as just part of women's care work and something women find easier to take than do men. Often the consequence is mental stress.

Unwanted sexual attention was also commonly experienced by the direct care workers in our survey, with nearly a third saying they experienced unwanted sexual attention on a daily or weekly basis and another 40 percent saying it happened at least once a month. Racism, too, was frequently reported by those working in long-term residential care. As a result of all these conditions and of their feelings of inadequacy, many workers leave work so preoccupied that they are unable to sleep. Nearly half said they sometimes or often lose sleep because of their work, and 18 percent told us this happens all or most of the time (Armstrong et al., 2009).

These various forms of violence take a toll on mental health, especially when workers' complaints are not taken seriously or, worse, as many we interviewed suggested, are dismissed as being caused by the worker herself. Moreover, the strain resulting from more limited forms of violence can contribute to worsening conditions, creating a vicious spiral of stress. In a survey of studies on caregivers' mental health, MacNeil et al. (2010) found that the stress of caregiving was not only likely to have an impact on the mental health of the provider, but to lead to angry and even physical assaults on those for whom they were providing care.

Control over work has been identified as a critical factor in mental health, but many of the women who provide care have little control over what they do, when, or for whom. Although women account for four out of five workers in health care, women do not, in the main, hold positions of power. Women are just half of the senior managers (CIHI, 2007), and those who provide the daily care often have little control over their work. In our research on long-term care, only a quarter of the Canadian workers said they could affect the planning of their day always or most of the time. Many women also have little choice about taking on unpaid care work, especially as services are cut back and as the health care system often assumes they will be available to do the work.

Mental health in health care work is also a women's issue because mental health is defined, experienced, and treated differently for women and men (Nasser, Baistow & Treasure, 2007). Women are more likely than men to seek help for mental distress, to be diagnosed with mental health problems, and to be hospitalized as a result. An analysis of more than 200 studies of unpaid caregivers concluded that, compared to men, women had higher levels of both depression and physical health problems (Pinquart & Sorensen, 2006). The consequences of mental health problems are also often different for women. A Statistics Canada study (Gilmour, 2008) reports, for instance, that "The risk of heart disease was significantly higher for women who had depression, but not for men" (p. 7). Luttik, Jaarsma, Lesman, Sanderman, and Hagedoorn (2009) found that women caring for those with heart failure are more likely than male care providers to experience negative health outcomes, including mental health issues.

Women are also the most likely to be thought of as bringing their personal and family problems to paid work, with the result that their mental health issues may be dismissed as simply a result of their other job or their sex. Katherine Lippel's (2007) work shows us that when women experience stress and mental illness, they are less likely than men to have their illness recognized as work related and less likely to be compensated as a result.

In short, the mental health of health care workers is a women's issue not only because most health care workers are women and because their conditions of work and of commitment differ from those of many men, but because women experience mental health differently than men, have their mental health issues treated differently than those of men, and have other work at home that exacerbates the stress.

## Understanding Women's Mental Health Problems at Work

As Mervat Nasser and colleagues (2007) explain in the introduction to their book *The Female Body in Mind*, we have to be cautious about interpreting the data on gender differences in mental health because they can hide assumptions about gender, mental health, and culture, as well as reflect the biases of the instruments dependent primarily on quantitative data. Nevertheless, as they go on to explain, "that an affinity exists between women and mental health problems is apparent not only in the statistics but also in cultural and historical representations or discursive constructions of 'women', 'women's bodies' and 'mental health' and 'illness'" (p. 6). Equally important, we are only beginning to understand the importance of the social and material locations of women and of the relational and power aspects of their work for women's mental health, as the participants in our workshop made clear. But we do know, as they also made clear, that women's work is changing in ways that can undermine mental health. "Studies on the impact of cost-reduction strategies report significant increases in staff depression, anxiety and emotional exhaustion among HCWs," according to Yassi and Hancock (2005, 35). They identified a number of critical factors, including "work overload, pressure at work, lack of participation in decision-making, poor social support, unsupportive leadership, lack of communication/feedback, staff shortages or unpredictable staffing, scheduling or long work hours and conflict between work and family demands" (p. 35). What is missing from this research is the role that gender plays and the consequences for women in particular.

We certainly heard about all of these factors from workshop participants, who came from a broad spectrum of academic, community, government, and health services. Karen Messing, an internationally recognized expert on women's occupational health, drew on her observational research to stress how workplace reorganization limits the possibility for the kinds of teamwork that support women in their jobs (Messing, 2008). Asked to conduct the research because of psychological distress among workers, the researchers found that the practices of shifting workers around and of hiring on a part-time and casual basis robbed women of support from colleagues. At the same time, the constant interruptions to their work added to their stress. In addition, the researchers found that both women and men brought fixed ideas about the division of labour and about who should do what and who did do what. There was an assumption that women would do more work in teams and would assign the harder physical labour to men, but neither assumption was validated by the researchers' observations. The very conflict between the assumptions and the reality contributed to the distress, leading the researchers to argue that stereotypes are also a factor.

Cathy Walker, a former director of health and safety at the Canadian Auto Workers, showed the impact of understaffing and little control on women's mental health. Women are struggling to make up for the care deficits, but leave work even after putting in unpaid overtime feeling that they did not do a good job. In our study of workers in long-term care (Armstrong et al., 2009, tables 19 and 23), Canadian women providing direct care were twice as likely as their Danish counterparts to say they felt inadequate all or most of the time, while 43 percent of the Canadian workers said they went home almost always feeling mentally exhausted, compared to only 8 percent of the Norwegian and Danish workers. These differences between Danish and Canadian health care workers suggest that mental exhaustion is not the inevitable result of the care work or the gender of the workers, but rather that the way work is organized is the most important factor in mental health. Moreover, health care workers may feel even more pressure than other workers to hide their mental health problems, given that they are supposed to be models of health and care (Preidt, 2010).

The same cost-reduction strategies that are having an impact on work in health care facilities are shaping the conditions of the growing number of women who do paid home care work. Although much of the stress faced by home care workers remains hidden in the household, Margaret Denton (2008) demonstrated how the pressure of for-profit managerial strategies mean women face high stress from low salaries, few benefits, and lack of job security, combined with the isolated nature of their jobs and the usual risks of care such as needle stick injuries. At the same time, though, she reminded us that the relational aspects of care work can promote mental health. Women gain real satisfaction from getting to know those for whom they provide care and from their expressed appreciation. Working alone can also have benefits in terms of developing a relationship with the person for whom they are providing care, even though working alone for women can also mean they are exposed to sexual and racial harassment.

Some women may be particularly at risk. As director of Rainbow Health Ontario, Anna Travers (2008) has witnessed the "environment of derision" that those who are lesbian, bisexual, and transgender too often face in their health care work. Indeed for a long time, same-sex relationships were taken as indicators of mental illness, and a residue of that notion remains in the way health care workers are treated by patients or other workers. The result can be increased anxiety, depression, substance abuse, and even suicide. Racism can have a similar impact and is often combined with sexism from both colleagues and patients (Jancur, 2008). For Aboriginal care providers, there is frequently the additional problem of working in isolated communities without peer support that could relieve the stress that comes both from being the only care provider and from facing the daily poverty and exploitation of those who need care (Johnson, 2008).

There are also important links between the stresses of paid and unpaid work. Given that many women do most of the domestic chores and care work at home while taking on paid care work, it is not surprising that women are more likely to feel stress from doing what is often referred to as balancing work and family life (Duxbury, Higgins & Schroeder, 2009). The stress may be felt particularly by women who work in health care not only because reforms have significantly increased their workloads and contributed to their feelings of inadequacy and lack of control, but also because they often go home to face similar kinds of demands there (Armstrong, Jansen, Connell & Jones, 2003). At the WHCR workshop, Cyndi Brannen (2008) offered an example of a shelter worker's stress and the relationship to her home:

> One of the hardest things is seeing children suffer and not being able to do anything about it ... my own kids are everything.... I would come back at the end of the day and e-mail my husband ... check the weather and tell him how to dress the kids for school tomorrow ... then think about the fact that those kids I was there to help might not live and nobody was thinking about whether or not they had warm jackets to wear.... I mean survival was their problem.

For women who provide unpaid care, the workload has increased with the closure of various residential care facilities just as the support provided by the state for care at home has declined. Based on interviews with such providers, Katherine Boydell (2008) reported that sourcing, organizing, and resourcing care created high levels of stress and interrupted their paid work. The women interviewed felt the pressure was on them as mothers, rather than on the fathers, to provide care. They became advocacy workers, fighting for services. Yet in spite of their long hours of work and the knowledge they gained from both providing care and advocating, they often had their expertise rejected or were dismissed as hysterical, creating yet more mental stress.

All this suggests that many health care reforms have had a profound impact on the mental health of women health care workers, making it more difficult for them to gain satisfaction from caring for others and more likely that they will face stress. Of course, the changing conditions of work are not the only factor explaining the mental health problems too many health care providers face. Mental health problems did not suddenly appear with the health care reforms of the 1990s, although it is clear that they have grown since then.

## The Questions Remaining

There can be little doubt that the mental health of women health care workers is a problem for them, for those who need care, and for the system as a whole. But many questions remain.

First, we need to try and sort out both those aspects of health care work that support good mental health for women and those aspects that undermine it. We also need to determine the aspects that can be changed and those that are inevitable in health care work.

Our comparative research on long-term care, for example, shows that Canadian long-term care workers are nearly six times more likely to experience daily violence as workers in Nordic countries, suggesting that there is little that is inevitable about violence in long-term care work (Armstrong et al., 2009, Figure 29).

Or consider the research indicating that, compared with nurses in women's health, pediatrics, and general practice, emergency nurses were 3.5 times as likely to use marijuana or cocaine; oncology and administration nurses were twice as likely to engage in binge drinking; and psychiatric nurses were most likely to smoke — clearly suggesting that work in health care can shape addictions among women (Statistics Canada, 2007). To what extent do these differences primarily reflect demands integral to care and to what extent do they reflect the way work is organized and gender is understood and practised? Even in the case of clearly necessary aspects of the work, such as 24-hour care, questions can be raised about how to organize the work to minimize the mental health consequences for women. A recent issue of *Perspectives on Labour and Income* (Williams, 2008), for instance, shows that women are significantly more likely than men to work rotating shifts that disrupt their body rhythms and family life. They are also more likely to work unpredictable shifts, with similar consequences.

Second, we need to try and sort out not only the specific issues for who does the paid and unpaid care work, but also the extent to which these are related to women's bodies. As Helen Malson and Mervat Nasser (2007) say in their provocatively titled chapter, "At Risk by Reason of Gender," "the answer to the question of why women appear more susceptible to mental health problems than men remains elusive" (p. 12). This does not mean asking if it is sex or if it is gender, expecting some clear division. As Fausto-Sterling (2005, 2006) makes clear, bodies cannot be separated from the relations and conditions in which they are embedded. However, we cannot leave out differences in bodies, including the differences among women's bodies, and in doing so must provide a gender analysis.

Such an analysis locates these bodies in the environments of paid and unpaid work, going beyond the simple task of collecting data by sex or comparing males and females (as much of the current research does if it considers gender at all) to understanding women's mental health within the context of their daily lives. It means beginning with the assumption that gender matters. It also means asking which women are affected in what ways. While it is useful to lump women together for the purposes of drawing attention to segregation, power, bodies, and other overall patterns, we need to know much more about the mental health consequences for women in different social, geographic, economic, occupational, and relational locations.

These are huge questions, but ones we need to address if we are to develop strategies that promote women's mental health and reduce costs not only to the individuals, their families, and to those for whom they provide care, but also for the system as a whole. We all have a vested interest in the mental health of health care workers.

## Note

1. CANSIM is the name of Statistics Canada's key socio-economic database. The data were calculated by Kate Laxer from the 2009 downloadable data.

## References

Armstrong, P., Armstrong, H. & Scott-Dixon, K. (2008). *Critical to care: The invisible women in health services.* Toronto: University of Toronto Press.

Armstrong, P., Banerjee, A., Szebehely, M., Armstrong, H., Daly, T. & Lafrance, S. (2009). *They deserve better: The long-term care experience in Canada and Scandinavia.* Ottawa: Canadian Centre for Policy Alternatives.

Armstrong, P., Jansen, I., Connell, E. & Jones, M. (2003). Assessing the impact of restructuring and work reorganization in long-term care. In P. Van Esterik (Ed.), *Head, heart, and hands: Partnerships for women's health in Canadian environments* (vol. 1, pp. 175–217). Toronto:

National Network on Environments and Women's Health.

Baines, D. (2006). Staying with people who slap you around: Gender, juggling responsibilities, and violence in paid (and unpaid) care work. *Gender, Work, and Organization 13*(2), 129–151.

Boydell, K. (2008, November). *Caringscapes: Mothering children with mental health disorders in rural and remote communities.* Presentation at the Workshop on the Mental Health of Women Health Care Workers, Women and Health Care Reform, and the BC Centre of Excellence for Women's Health, Vancouver.

Brannen, C. (2006). Women's unpaid caregiving and stress. *Centres of Excellence for Women's Health Research Bulletin 5*(1), 12–13. Retrieved from http://www.cewh-cesf.ca/PDF/RB/bulletin-vol5no1EN.pdf

Brannen, C. (2008, November). *Invisible warriors, hidden wounds, secondary traumatic stress, and women caregivers.* Presentation at the Workshop on the Mental Health of Women Health Care Workers, Women and Health Care Reform, and the BC Centre of Excellence for Women's Health, Vancouver.

Campbell, Andrea. (2010) Annotated Bibliography on the Mental Health Of Women Health Care Workers http://www.womenand-healthcarereform.ca/publications/ mentalHealthWomenHealth-CareWorkersAnnotBiblio.pdf

Canadian Institute for Health Information (CIHI). (2007). *Canada's health care providers, 2007.* Ottawa: CIHI.

Canadian Institute for Health Information (CIHI). (2008). *Health personnel trends, 1995–2004* (Appendix F). Retrieved from http://secure.cihi.ca/cihiweb/products/Health _Personnel_Trend_1995-2004_e.pdf

Cochrane, J., Goering, P.N. & Rogers, J.M. (1997). The mental health of informal caregivers in Ontario: An epidemiological survey. *American Journal of Public Health 87*(12), 2002–2007.

Cranswick, K. & Dosman, D. (2008) Eldercare: What we know today *Canadian Social Trends*, 47-57.

Denton, M. (1997). The linkages between informal and formal care of the elderly. *Canadian Journal on Aging/La Revue Canadienne du Vieillissment 16*(1), 17–37.

Denton, M. (2008, November). *Unraveling the impact of care work.* Panel presentation at the Workshop on the Mental Health of Women

Health Care Workers, Women and Health Care Reform, and the BC Centre of Excellence for Women's Health, Vancouver.

Dhawan, S. (1998). *Caregiving stress and acculturation in East Indian immigrants: Caring for their elders.* Unpublished doctoral dissertation, Queen's University, Kingston.

Dion Stout, M. (2008, November). *Weaving death and dance baskets and unraveling space and place concepts.* Keynote presentation at the Workshop on the Mental Health of Women Health Care Workers, Women and Health Care Reform, and the BC Centre of Excellence for Women's Health, Vancouver.

Duxbury, L., Higgins, C. & Schroeder, B. (2009, January). *Balancing paid work and caregiver responsibilities: A closer look at family caregivers in Canada.* Retrieved from http://www.cprn.org/documents/51061_EN.pdf

European Union (EU). (2003). *Gender issues in health and safety at work.* Luxembourg: European Agency for Safety and Health at Work.

Fausto-Sterling, A. (2005). "The bare bones of sex: Part I, Sex and gender." *Signs 30*(2), 1491–1527.

Fausto-Sterling, A. (2006). "Bare bones of sex: Part II, Race and bones." *Social Studies of Science 38*(5), 657–694.

Gilmour, H. (2008). Depression and the risk of heart disease. *Health Reports 19*(3), 7–17.

Haegedoorn, M., Sanderman, R., Buunk, B.P. (2002). Failing in spousal caregiving: The "identity-relevant stress" hypothesis to explain sex differences in caregiver distress. *British Journal of Health Psychology 7*(4), 481–492.

Jancur, A. (2008, November). *Social locations.* Panel presentation at the Workshop on the Mental Health of Women Health Care Workers, Women and Health Care Reform, and the BC Centre of Excellence for Women's Health, Vancouver.

Johnson, E. (2008, November). *Social locations.* Panel presentation at the Workshop on the Mental Health of Women Health Care Workers, Women and Health Care Reform, and the BC Centre of Excellence for Women's Health, Vancouver.

Kirby, M. (2008). Mental health in Canada: Out of the shadows forever. *Canadian Medical Association Journal 178*(10).

Koehoorn, M., Ibrahim, S., Hertzman, C., Ostry, A. & Brown, J. (2009). Regions, hospitals, and health outcomes over time: A multi-level analysis of repeat prevalence among a cohort of health-care workers. *Health and Place 15*(4), 1046–1057.

Lippel, K. (2007). Work and mental health. *International Journal of Law and Psychiatry 30*(4–5), 269–457.

Luttik, M.L., Jaarsma, T., Lesman, I., Sanderman, R. & Hagedoorn, M. (2009). Quality of life in partners with congestive heart failure: Gender and involvement in care. *Journal of Advanced Nursing 65*(7), 1442–1451.

MacNeil, G., Kosberg, I.J., Durkin, D.W., Dooley, W.K., DeCoster, J. & Williamson, G.M. (2010). Caregiver mental health and potentially harmful caregiving behavior: The central role of caregiver anger. *The Gerontologist 50*(1), 76–86.

Malson, H. & Nasser, M. (2007). At risk by reason of gender. In M. Nasser, K. Baistow & J. Treasure (Eds.), *The female body in mind: The interface between the female body and mental health* (pp. 3–16). New York: Routledge.

Meshefedjian, G., McCusker, J., Bellavance, F. & Baumgarten, M. (1998). Factors associated with symptoms of depression among informal caregivers of demented elders in the community. *The Gerontologist 38*(2), 247–253.

Messing, K. (1998). *One-eyed science: Occupational health and women workers*. Philadelphia: Temple University Press.

Messing, K. (2008, November). *The importance of supporting teamwork for the well-being of health-care workers*. Presentation at the Workshop on the Mental Health of Women Health Care Workers, Women and Health Care Reform, and the BC Centre of Excellence for Women's Health, Vancouver.

Nasser, M., Baistow, K. & Treasure, J. (Eds.). (2007). *The female body in mind: The interface between the female body and mental health*. New York: Routledge.

Pinquart, M. & Sorensen, S. (2006). Gender differences in caregiver stressors, social resources, and health: An updated meta-analysis. *The Journals of Gerontology: Series B 61*(1), 33–45.

Preidt, R. (2010, January 30). Workers fear stigma of seeking mental health care. *Healthday News.* Retrieved from http://www.medi-cinenet.com/script/main/ art.asp?articlekey=112841

Public Health Agency of Canada. (2002). *A report on mental illness in Canada.* Retrieved from http://www.phac-aspc.gc.ca/publicat/miic-mmac/chap_2-eng.php

Scientific Advisory Committee to the Global Business and Economic Roundtable on Addiction and Mental Health. (2002). *Mental health and substance use at work: Perspectives from research and implications for leaders.* Retrieved from http://www .mentalhealthroundtable. ca/jan_2003/mentalhealth2_nov11_021.pdf

Shields, M. & Wilkins, K. (2006). *Findings from the 2005 National Survey of Work and Health of Nurses.* Ottawa: Ministry of Industry.

Statistics Canada. (2007). *2005 National Survey of the Work and Health of Nurses.* Ottawa: Health Canada.

Statistics Canada. (2009). Work absence rates. Retrieved from http://www.statcan.gc.ca/pub/71-211-x/71-211-x2010000-eng.pdf

Statistics Canada. (2010). *Employment by major industry groups, season-ally adjusted, by province (monthly).* Retrieved from http://www40. statcan.gc.ca/ l01/cst01/labr67a-eng.htm

Travers, A. (2008, November). *Social locations.* Panel presentation at the Workshop on the Mental Health of Women Health Care Workers, Women and Health Care Reform, and the BC Centre of Excellence for Women's Health, Vancouver.

Trinkoff, A.M. & Storr, C.L. (1998). Substance use among nurses: Differ-ences between specialties. *American Journal of Public Health 88*(4), 581–585.

Walker, C. (2008, November). *Chronically caregiving.* Panel presenta-tion at the Workshop on the Mental Health of Women Health Care Workers, Women and Health Care Reform, and the BC Centre of Excellence for Women's Health, Vancouver.

Williams, C. (2008). Work-life balance of shift workers. *Perspectives on Labour and Income 9*(8), 3–16.

Yassi, A. & Hancock, T. (2005). Patient safety: Building a culture of safety to improve healthcare worker and patient well-being. *Healthcare Quarterly 8*(Special Issue), 3208.

CHAPTER 9

# Woman-Defined Quality Care

PAT ARMSTRONG, MADELINE BOSCOE, BARBARA CLOW,
KAREN R. GRANT, NANCY GUBERMAN, BETH JACKSON,
ANN PEDERSON, AND KAY WILLSON

## Introduction

Time and quality in health care have been issues of concern, not
only in Canada but throughout the Western world. For example, Ujjal Dosanjh (2004), the then Canadian minister of Health,
emphasized "the timeliness and quality of health care services"
in his introduction to a report on the state of the health system.
Like many others, however, this report considers time exclusively
in terms of time waiting for health care services while quality is
defined in terms of hospitalization rates and of patients' satisfaction with services (Health Canada, 2004). This is only one report
among many, but it reflects dominant themes in both the research
literature and policy fields (Jackson, 2003). Yet those interviewed
by the Women and Health Care Reform team about their definitions of quality care were at least as concerned about time in care
and for care—that is, about appropriate time allocated to respond
to their needs and about care providers having enough time to
do so. For these women, quality and time are integrally linked
through the process of care. This chapter explores how the women

we interviewed across Canada define time issues in quality care, and the implications for how quality is understood. It differs from the other chapters, which offer an analysis of secondary sources, providing data on a neglected area and an example of doing primary, gender-based research.

## Our Research Question

Our research question was both complex and simple: How do women define quality in health care? It was simple in the sense of being direct and focused. It was complex both in the sense that "women" are not a simple, single group, and that quality is an ambiguous, multifaceted concept. As Kassirer explained in the *New England Journal of Medicine*:

> Underlying the expectation that physicians, health plans, and other organizations will soon be competing on the basis of the quality as well as the cost of medical care is the fundamental assumption that we know what quality is and how to measure it, monitor it, and ensure it. This is a proposition devoutly to be wished, and one to which millions of dollars will be devoted. But how accurate is it? (1993, 1263)

Given this complexity, it is not surprising that the responses to our question were wide-ranging. This chapter focuses on one common theme that emerged — namely, time.

## Conceptual Grounds

Our research for this project is guided by the literature on feminist political economy (Armstrong et al., 2002; Doyal, 1995; Grant et al., 2004; Messing, 1998; Petchesky, 2003), on the social determinants of health (Evans, Barer & Marmor, 1994; Marmot & Wilkinson,

1999; Marmot, 2004; Raphael, 2009; Robertson, 1998), on quality (see Jackson, 2003), and on time (Hochschild, 2000; Postone, 1996; Weston, 2002; Whipp, Adam & Sabelis, 2002). Chapter 1 introduces our theoretical approach, but we would like to stress the basic assumptions that are particularly relevant to our research on how women define quality care.

First, we assume that gender matters. Gender is understood as a socially constructed relationship that shapes not only our economic and social possibilities, but also the ways our bodies develop, are experienced, and treated. Women's experiences can be taken into account in their own right, and not only in comparison to those of men.

Second, we assume that there are differences among women related to their specific social, economic, and physical locations and relations, differences that often matter in how care is experienced and delivered. Because we assume that gender is socially constructed, we also assume that biology does not produce two genders that are shaped by and experienced in distinct, dichotomous ways. Moreover, women participate in the health care system as patients, providers, and decision-makers, both distinct and overlapping aspects of women's lives that also influence their experiences.

And third, we assume that women speaking from their own experiences can tell us a great deal about care and should be consulted about how they define quality in health care. As Dubé, Ferland, and Moskowitz (2003, 4) point out in their discussion of challenges for health research, real progress in managing health will come from an "understanding of day-to-day caring from both the patients and the provider's perspectives."

The social determinants of health literature leads us to assume that health care is about much more than technical interventions through surgery and drugs (Armstrong & Armstrong, 2010). We go beyond the usual approach to the social determinants literature, however, in assuming that the same factors that influence health outside health care also influence health within care. This means that social support and working conditions, for example, are at least as important to determining the quality of care as they are to determining health overall. It also means that context matters.

Our survey (Jackson, 2003) of the literature on quality revealed a focus on structural components, processes, and outcomes. In general, these three aspects tend to be treated as independent variables, with researchers studying either resources, or interpersonal relations, or mortality rates, for example. Given our assumptions about the centrality of the determinants of health, including gender, within health care, we also assume that all three aspects of quality are related to each other in continuing and complex ways.

Finally, we looked to the literature on time to include our interest in the ways that care processes are reorganized through health care reforms. In health care, labour is the major expense. Labour time is money spent on care. The increasing emphasis on cost saving and on for-profit methods of managing health care has meant a focus on time for care and time in care, with providers spending less time with each care recipient and people being sent home "quicker and sicker" from services. Time is thus a significant component in care.

## Our Research Methods

Our methods were shaped by these assumptions. We interviewed 145 women in 26 different focus groups. These semi-structured interviews were conducted in the Atlantic provinces, Quebec, Ontario, Manitoba, Saskatchewan, and British Columbia, with groups designed to capture a broad range of women. Each group was organized with particular social, economic, and geographical locations in mind: young, middle-aged, and old; immigrant, First Nations, and Canadian-born; lesbian, queer, bisexual, and heterosexual; street-involved women with addictions and university students; poor and economically comfortable; women of size; mothers and service providers; urban and rural dwelling women; with some groups more varied in membership.

We chose focus groups as our data-collection technique for several reasons.

First, the focus group method is consistent with our theoretical approach as it allows us to investigate "situated knowledge"— that is, how women's multiple roles (as patients, paid and unpaid providers, and decision-makers) and locations (socially, economically, culturally, physically, and in terms of age, ability, and sexual orientation) influence their perceptions and experiences. Second, focus groups by their very nature are intended to stimulate discussion. By using this method we were able to bring together groups of women to carry out a dialogue about their experiences of health care. Rather than attending only to what individual women had to say, we were able to benefit from the more participatory nature of focus groups, which allow individuals with common experiences to stimulate one another. In short, the focus groups made it possible for us to identify shared experiences and information, and the group discussions also served as a "reality check" for those in attendance. That we found similar experiences across many different groups involving a wide variety of women's experiences similarly allowed us to arrive at some common understandings about women's encounters with the health care system, while exploring the importance of intersectionality at the same time. Finally, the focus group method made it possible to gather accounts from a large number of women in an efficient way. The loss of privacy and personalized attention that women would have had in an individual interview were more than made up for by the captivating and engaging discussions that we had with women from across the country.

Beginning with a semi-structured interview guide, we prompted discussions about their experiences with and in health care; about what makes health care good or bad; what defines care as quality care; what makes the issue of quality health care a women's issue; and women's perspectives on current indicators of quality in health care.

Once the focus groups were completed, each interview was

transcribed verbatim. We used *N6*, a qualitative data analysis software program, to conduct our analyses. All transcripts were coded based upon an initial set of coding categories and subcategories derived from a review of the interview transcripts. Then, taking each of the coding categories individually, we developed our analyses accordingly. Over several meetings of the team, the coding and analyses were cross-checked to ensure that we had been systematic and comprehensive in our approach to the data.

Such a method involves developing an analysis in the process of coding and reading the data. It also means that rather than separately presenting the data to be analyzed, we combined our findings with our discussion.

## It's About Time

In every group, time emerged as a critical issue without prompting from us. While some talked about time in terms of waiting for services, waiting times for tests, hips and for eyes or cancer and heart care were not the most frequently mentioned time or quality issues. Rather, these women emphasized the time for care and the time in care.

A low-income woman in Saskatchewan summed up her view of what defined quality care by saying simply "time," while a middle-class Quebec woman expanded somewhat on the same theme, saying, "For well-being, you need people who take time." A participant in a group made up of providers in a women's clinic who had just assessed their own organization summed up the discussion by saying that "all these processes take time. That's the big factor in providing quality care."

Women want providers who take the time to understand them as people rather than as pieces to be fixed. In Atlantic Canada, a doctor was described as excellent in a group of daycare mothers because "she'll sit down with me for half an hour if I need to ask questions and depending on what I need." A young graduate student likes her doctor "because when I go in, she sits down and looks at my chart and, you know, she asks me what I'm up to now and stuff like that. So she takes the time to work with me." In Quebec, an injured worker reports positively on "this one doctor I went to after having many experiences with others. I walked in there, he sits me down and he asks you completely what your problem is. He doesn't want to whisk you out of his office ... and give you a prescription." A Manitoba woman with chronic health conditions speaks of a provider who answered her questions "thoroughly. She wasn't rushing me." A Saskatchewan woman said quality care is

> When you really have time to talk about what is going on in your life or what's changed since you last saw them and they take an interest and they know you by name and they take the time to understand who you are or where you are coming from.

And in BC, a young woman offered midwives as an example of good care. "Every time I questioned, even if it was a dumb question, they would readily answer and let me know what's going on and not to worry. Calm down. Everything's normal. They were there with me at the birth for a good 12 hours."

The reports of positive experiences with providers taking the time to understand the whole person contrasted with the many who talked about being rushed and having no time to have their issues understood. Women reported facing extreme time limits for interaction with providers, as well as a limit on the number of issues they could raise. Listen to an Ontario lesbian woman:

> I think that some of the doctors, and I've heard my mom say this too, is that you can only go and you can only deal with one thing at a time. I've heard my partner say it too. And it's completely ridiculous. Like what is this only one problem at a time? First of all, we're all busy. Why can't I talk about

three things? I haven't got, you know two other times to come back.... That's not treating you as a whole person.... You don't separate mind and body so how would you even be okay with asking me about my kidneys and ignoring my heart? How can you talk about one system in isolation? It's completely ludicrous. So I mean I feel very obviously passionate about that, that we're treated as a whole person and not rushed out the door.

It is about more than feeling good, although the literature on the determinants of health tell us social support is critical to health. For this woman, the severe time pressure not only fails to give her an accurate diagnosis, but also uses her time inappropriately as well. A middle-aged Saskatchewan woman tells a similar story:

Like in my doctor's office now, there is a note that says your physician is only paid to see you for 10 minutes. Please make sure that when you see the physicians, you're only going to discuss one or two things.... So I think it's in the patients', and those health professionals'—those health care workers'—interest for things to be changed so that it's more focused on improving quality of care, allowing those people to spend more time with patients.

So does a senior in Quebec. A young Manitoba woman talks about efficiency "where doctors are required to have so many appointments per hour that people are basically shoved in and out the door." While there has always been a limit on how much time any provider can give, women report experiencing increasing time pressures and a changed attitude on the part of providers. A BC woman described her doctor of 15 years with whom she used to be able to "really take [her] time."

But in recent years I noticed like, it's like, I have a time limit. And I go in there and then before I feel totally satisfied in terms of talking about my problems, it's like, that's it. Right? So I don't know if it's a change in the system or what but that's my sort of experience with her.

In Ontario, one of the senior women says she feels as if she is in an assembly line, a feeling she shares with many of those we interviewed. But the limited time means

> if you go in with some problem and suddenly it comes up that your marriage is falling apart or there's some major issue in your life, you don't have time to talk with your physician about that because the time has ended and you'll have to make another appointment. It's very, very bad.

Both the patient and the provider have to take more time through another appointment at the expense of the system and the women. In a Saskatchewan group, a woman succinctly summarized the issue, saying "the five minutes in the office might be efficient for them but it's not efficient for the user."

The failure to take the time to understand the whole person has consequences both for the women who seek care and for the system as a whole. Health issues can be missed, women say, because the provider does not have time to investigate things like breast cancer, for example.

> I once had an annual check-up, which the doctor gets paid a certain amount for. And there were a number of things I knew he was supposed to be doing, including the breast exam, which he skipped because he said he didn't have time.

This lack of a prescribed breast examination would not show up in the data on quality because, "according to the health care system, I already had my annual check-up, so I had to go without certain tests that year." As a BC immigrant woman put it, "they're trying to be too efficient and they don't really take into account everything that is going on and they don't take the time to really see what is involved or what is medical." For those with cultural, language, and economic issues, even more time is required to draw out the women's concerns and to communicate results.

Health issues can also be missed because the provider does not have time to make the patient feel comfortable and allow her to explain her problem in context. A young Ontario woman feels uncomfortable with doctors, and a short time frame means "they're really not going to try and draw stuff out of me because they don't have time to talk either."

Short visits also mean there is little time for doctors to explain information about their diagnosis and treatment. The lack of explanation can increase stress levels, as well as prevent patients from following through appropriately on tests, drugs, or treatments. It can also mean that women who take family members to medical appointments do not have time to learn about appropriate care. This was the case for a BC immigrant woman who visited the doctor with her mother "for like two minutes. And she said 'Yeah, all right, okay, bye.' And I was like, 'Okay, I still have more questions' but she had already walked out the door."

A young Ontario woman spoke about being diagnosed with a heart condition by a care provider who did

> not explain what the consequences are, not explain; not explain what the chances are.... You would probably be anxious for that month anyway but you would have been less anxious about it [if it was explained]. Like that's a pretty big thing to lay on somebody and then sort of leave five minutes later.

Ontario seniors provided several examples of limited time for communication, with negative consequences for their health. A woman with long-term disabilities talked about the doctor's failure to "listen to what's working and what isn't" from the patient's perspective. This failure to communicate and to listen results in stress for the patient, they said. It also means costs for the system.

> You don't have time. It's always just a few minutes with them. You don't feel comfortable so you need to go to somebody else to be able to deal with the emotional, physical issues that you're going through, [somebody] that you can talk to and feel comfortable with and trust.

A number of the women in the focus groups mentioned short appointments as a factor in the increasing reliance on drugs. A middle-aged Saskatchewan woman said, "You wait there for a good hour and they spend like five minutes with you and give you a prescription and send you on your way." According to a Quebec senior, "they don't even take enough time to talk to you. You would complain about something and [they say] 'Okay, take this pill, come back in two weeks if it doesn't work or you have side effects.'"

This rush through care, with short appointments and little time in the care encounter, costs women more than just additional medical problems. A telling example was provided by a group of senior women. They spoke about the well-baby clinics that were available to them in the 1960s.

> I never needed a pediatrician. I would walk over, with a buggy full of babies, to the church where there was a pediatrician that was being paid by the government. There were psychologists that were testing the kids to see if they were ready for school. There was a nutritionist discussing diet with me. There were people who were watching how the children interacted with each other. Our appointments would be up to two hours. They were absolutely exceptional. They got all their immunizations and if there were any behavioural problems, you could speak to the psychologist and they would help you through this.

The point is not only that her children got care in ways that considered them as whole people and combined multiple assessments and interventions. And it is not only that such an approach allowed health problems to be prevented or caught before they developed into serious issues. It is also that a woman had to make only one appointment for all her children and their health issues. This contrasts sharply with the women who complained that with doctors limiting visits to one patient and one problem, they were constantly taking time off work to arrange for their children's care. This is a women's issue because it is mainly women who take children to care, even though the overwhelming majority of women now work for pay and have employment hours similar to those of men.

It should be noted, however, that these women did not expect unlimited time for care or instant service. As an Ontario university student put it, her family doctor is

> Really, really excellent. I mean when you go in and see her, even though you have an appointment, you expect to wait between half an hour and an hour. But you know that when it's your turn that she'll give you as much time as you need for whatever you need and that's pretty rare.

When we asked if this was more important than getting in on time, she responded,

> Yes. I'd rather know that when I get in, ... I'm going to feel like I, you know, I'm not being rushed through, that I'm not being passed over, that my concerns are not being dismissed.

Similarly, a young street woman says that in the clinic she visits, "everyone usually waits like half an hour. The most is an hour that I wait but I don't mind because my doctors are good. They know what they are doing." She goes on to say that she gets "personal attention" and time.

Many of the other women, however, confirmed that such experiences were rare. More common were long waits that led to very short encounters, leaving the women feeling frustrated by their care. Rather than unlimited time, these women talked about time required for care. Those we interviewed wanted time that would allow providers to understand their specific health issues, to listen, to encourage, to explain, to combine issues in a way that deals with whole people.

This leads to a final point about their expectations and understanding of quality. Although they talk about good and bad provider s, they are much more likely to attribute the fault to reforms in the health care system than to the individual provider. It was common for women to follow their comments on being rushed through the doctor's office with explanations beyond the individual. For example, after complaining that "the doctors don't listen and things," a young mother explains that the doctor has no choice because there are so many patients needing care. In the same interview, another woman added,

> if I was a doctor I'd find that extremely stressful to know you have more patients that you need to see. So subconsciously you're going to try and rush. Rush. I would.

Similarly, an injured Quebec worker qualified her critique: "I'm not saying that they don't want to listen but they simply don't have the time. The waiting room is filled up." According to a Manitoba woman, "doctors are required to have so many appointments per hour, people are basically shoved in and out the door. They don't have time to spend with the people who need it," while an Ontario university student who worked in health care maintained that "if you didn't churn out 80 people a day you were slow." She went on to say this pressure for speed encourages providers to see patients as a nuisance and to dismiss their symptoms.

These women were particularly sympathetic to the nurses who are expected to provide the daily care in facilities and homes.

A Métis woman was especially eloquent about the conditions nurses face and the impact on the quality of care they can provide, although her comments were echoed in the other interviews. She said,

> What's very clear when you're in the hospital is that the doctors are essentially not around and the day-to-day care is provided by the aides and the nurses and what you really want when you are in the hospital, you want some of that person's time. And when you have that person's attention, you need that person to be able to listen to you for a while. And the nurses now, in my experience, they all wear running shoes because that's all they do all day is they run. And they feel terrible with the quality of care they're giving because they literally can't spend the time with anybody. So I think it's in the patient's interest for things to be changed, so there is more focus on improving the quality of care allowing those people to spend time with patients. Whereas right now, it's all about saving money and reducing, you know, hospital expenditures to the barest amount possible.

Speaking of what she saw while attending to a hospitalized patient for whom she was responsible, a young Ontario woman who helped care for an elderly neighbour reported that

> Other people that were there that didn't have support, they just didn't get it, you know, because the health care workers didn't have the time to give it. And how depressed and angry and upset they were at being in the hospital … and just not having the support. And it made a huge difference…. If you focus more and more on tasks and at the same time the people who are there are sicker … more of that is going to happen if you don't have people around.

In the same focus group, another woman talked about the lack of cleaners and other staff, as well as nurses, and her concern that the people she saw in hospitals did not get bathed as frequently as necessary to be comfortable.

> Like it's almost inhumane. Even more than being dirty and stuff is sitting there in your bed. You know, people that were told they were not going to walk again lying in their beds just crying and having no one come for hours.... Or else people are being really angry ... and yelling and yelling 'cause they're so upset.... And the hospital staff are in a frenzy themselves 'cause they're burned out.

Senior women reported a similar lack of time for care, with similar consequences for the patients. "A lot of these people are very alone.... They are desperate for somebody just to come in and say 'Good morning. How are you? We care about you.' They're not given the time." This group also provided an example of a disabled person not getting care "because they are not given the time to spend with their patients or their clients, call them what you will."

But these women were also concerned about the consequences for the nurses. According to a First Nations woman, her nurse exploded, yelling at a patient, because "she just couldn't deal with any more stress." While she explained this in terms of "a big shortage," the group went on to say there was no shortage of nurses, just a shortage of full-time jobs.

Lack of time for care by paid providers means women have to take the time to be a patient advocate or an unpaid caregiver. An elderly Ontario woman reported that her friends "may or may not eat and I just go right to the hospital to make sure that somebody is there to look after them and be a patient advocate for them." Another woman in that seniors' group knew a patient who did not get bathed because the staff "were overworked" so she had to do it.

In sum, these women see time in care and for care as key to quality. They want time to explain, to be understood. They want providers to take the time to treat them as whole people, listening, prompting, explaining, and exchanging information. They do not see this time as a luxury—a frill—but rather as critical to care. For many, taking time means being "treated with respect." They are quite prepared to wait a reasonable time for care if there is time for them when their turn comes. They see the lack of time for care as mainly a product of reforms, rather than as a result of poor providers.

The literature on the determinants of health reinforces their view of time. Social support and empowerment are critical components in health, so it is not surprising that they should also be critical in care. The literature also suggests that medical errors are rising along with time pressure, just as these women say. In addition, women want time in care to be organized in order to take their time pressures into account. Most women work for pay and most women take primary responsibility not only for their own health, but for that of their families. Quality care would recognize these pressures and accommodate them in the organization of care time. Too many women suffer from what a young Quebec woman called a "poverty of time" along with economic poverty. As a result, "you know, you don't have time to be scheduling and running around and stuff like that."

# Conclusion

As Dubé, Ferland, and Moskowitz (2003, 3) make clear, efforts to improve quality through evidence-based practice initiatives have not paid much attention to "the more human aspects of care, including the interpersonal and emotional processes that are at play between patient and the provider in each episode of care." There was some variation among women in different social locations, but all the women we interviewed said time in and for care are critical components in quality. Regardless of their social, economic, or physical location, they want the time they need to explain, to understand, to link their health issues to each other, as well as to the context of their own lives. They want providers to have more time, which means they want more human resources for care and different management of care. They want an emphasis on the interpersonal and emotional aspects of care because it leads to better outcomes.

Our purpose in asking women how they defined quality care was to contribute to the general move toward evidence-informed decision-making and quality improvement in ways that take women's experiences into account. The emphasis participants put on care—this desire for time—may seem obvious, but it has not been obvious in policy documents on improving the quality of care. Indeed, the opposite is the case. The focus is on reducing time in and for care, a strategy that these women say undermines the quality of their care.

# References

Armstrong, P. & Armstrong, H. (2010). *Wasting away: The undermining of Canadian health care.* Toronto: Oxford University Press.

Armstrong, P., et al. (2002). *Exposing privatization: Women and health care reform in Canada.* Aurora: Garamond.

Brannen, J. (2005). Time and the negotiation of work-family boundaries. *Time and Society 14*(1), 113–131.

Dosanjh, U. (2004). Message from the minister of health. *Healthy Canadians: A federal report on comparable health indicators.* Ottawa: Health Canada.

Doyal, L. (1995). *What makes women sick: Gender and the political economy of health.* New Brunswick: Rutgers University Press.

Dubé, L., Ferland, G. & Moskowitz, D.S. (2003). Integrating the art and science of care into the everyday delivery of health services: Challenges for research and practice. In L. Dubé, G. Ferland & D.S. Moskowitz (Eds.), *Emotional and interpersonal dimensions of health services.* Montreal: McGill-Queen's University Press.

Evans, R.G., Barer, M.L. & Marmor, T.R. (Eds.). (1994). *Why are some people healthy and others not? The determinants of population health.* New York: Aldine De Gruyter.

Grant, Karen, et al. (2004). *Caring for/caring about: Women and unpaid caregiving in Canada.* Aurora: Garamond Press.

Health Canada. (2004). Healthy Canadians: A Federal Report on Comparable Health Indicators 2004 http://www.hc-sc.gc.ca/hcs-sss/pubs/system-regime/2004-fed-comp-indicat/index-eng.php#a1

Health Council of Canada. (2005). Wait times and access. Background paper to accompany *Health care renewal in Canada: Accelerating change.* Toronto: Health Council of Canada.

Hochschild, A.R. (2000). *The time bind.* New York: Henry Holt.

Jackson, B.E. (2003). Situating epidemiology. Gender Perspectives on Health and Medicine: Key Themes. Advances in Gender Research Series. Volume 7. Marcia Texler Segal, Vasilikie Demos and Jennie Kronenfeld (eds.) Greenwich, CN: JAI Press.

Kassirer, J.P. (1993). The quality of care and the quality of measuring it. *New England Journal of Medicine* 329(17), 1263–1265.

Marmot, M. & Wilkinson, R.C. (1999). *Social determinants of health.* New York: Oxford University Press.

Marmot, M. (2004). *The status syndrome: How social standing affects our health and longevity.* London: Henry Holt.

Messing, K. (1998). *One-eyed science: Occupational health and women workers.* Philadelphia: Temple University Press.

Petchesky, R.P. (2003). *Global prescriptions gendering health and human rights.* London: Zed Books.

Postone, M. (1996). *Time, labor, and social domination.* Cambridge: Cambridge University Press.

Raphael, D. (Ed.). (2009). *Social determinants of health: Canadian perspectives.* Toronto: Canadian Scholars' Press Inc.

Robertson, A. (1998). Shifting discourses on health in Canada: From health promotion to population health. *Health Promotion International* 13(2), 155–166.

Weston, K. (2002). *Gender in real time.* New York: Routledge.

Whipp, R., Adam, B. & Sabelis, I. (2002). *Making time: Time and management in modern organizations.* Oxford: Oxford University Press.

CHAPTER 10

# Women and Private Health Insurance

ALISON JENKINS JAYMAN AND KAY WILLSON

## Introduction

Who pays for care matters to women. Women make greater use of health care services than men, accounting for 55 percent of provincial and territorial health expenditures in Canada (Canadian Institute for Health Information, 2010). In part, women's greater use of health services can be attributed to their reproductive health care needs, their higher rates of chronic disease, and their longer lifespan, as well as to the way they are treated by the system and their responsibility for taking children to care services. Women use health services more, but have fewer financial resources to cover health care costs (Forget et al., 2005). Women, on average, earn less than men and face higher rates of poverty. Women's lower income, combined with higher demand for health care, means that individual health expenditures pose a greater financial risk to women than to men (Rustgi, Doty & Collins, 2009). Since private health insurance is designed to protect people from the financial risks of health care costs, it is an issue of particular importance to women.

Women are also the majority of paid and unpaid providers of health care. The health sector is a major source of female employment, and health care financing has an impact on the conditions of women's paid and unpaid work. Given the gendered nature of health care and the gender gap in income, it is clear that changes in health care financing "can affect men and women differently, as a consequence of their different positions as users and producers of health care" (Ostlin, 2005, 4). Yet changes in health care financing and other health reforms are seldom examined through a gender lens.

This chapter focuses on the gendered consequences of one particular area of health reform—the expansion of private health insurance as a source of health care financing. The privatization of health care financing is part of a much broader pattern of privatization in health reform, a pattern that has been shown to have important and often negative consequences for women (Armstrong et al., 2002).

Concerns about the rising costs of health care have put the issue of health financing on the public policy agenda. Proposals to expand the role of private health insurance have attracted interest in Canada and around the world. In considering these proposals, it is important to ask how the expansion of private health insurance will affect women as a group and particular groups of women. To what extent does private insurance offer women protection against the financial costs of health care? How does private insurance affect women's access to care? To explore these questions, we examine some of the literature on gender and private health insurance in Canada, the United States, and other OECD countries. Our discussion builds on and updates earlier work on this topic produced for Women and Health Care Reform (WHCR) (see Jenkins, 2007). Before turning to the evidence, we provide an overview of health care financing in Canada and the growing debate over private health insurance.

# Health Care Financing in Canada

According to the Canadian Institute for Health Information, total expenditures for health care in Canada will reach almost $192 billion in 2010. Approximately 70 percent of health care is financed by the public sector, 13 percent is financed by private health insurance, and 17 percent is financed by other private expenditures, primarily out-of-pocket payments (Canadian Institute for Health Information, 2010). The level of public health financing in Canada is comparable to that in other advanced industrial countries, but the level of private health insurance financing is much higher than most. Within OECD countries, public spending accounts for 72 percent of total health expenditures, and private health insurance pays for only 6.3 percent (Colombo & Tapay, 2004a). The main exception is the United States, where private health insurance plays a much greater role and accounts for 35 percent of total health expenditures (Colombo & Tapay, 2004a).

Today nearly all Canadians are protected by medicare, a system of universal public health insurance financed by general taxation. Medicare provides comprehensive coverage of medically necessary hospital and physician services. Although each province and territory administers its own system of public health insurance, they all must adhere to the basic principles of medicare as defined in the *Canada Health Act*. This law, which can be seen to build on the foundations of the 1957 *Hospital Insurance and Diagnostic Services Act* and the 1966 *Medical Care Act*, was passed by the federal government in 1984. It requires that provincial health insurance programs be universal, comprehensive, accessible, portable, and publicly administered in order to qualify for federal funding.

In the *Canada Health Act*, the criterion of *universality* requires that all residents have access to public health care insurance and insured services under the same terms and conditions. *Comprehensiveness* demands that provinces actually insure services that are defined as "insured health services." *Accessibility* involves ensuring that all insured people have reasonable and uniform access to insured health services. This means that no one may be discriminated against on the basis of factors such as income, age, or health status. *Portability* requires that provinces cover "insured health services" for those temporarily absent from their province of residence. In order to satisfy the criterion of *public administration*, each provincial health care insurance plan must be administered and operated on a non-profit basis by a public authority that is accountable to the provincial government.

Under this system, every Canadian can seek emergency care, visit a doctor, access diagnostic services, be treated by a variety of medical specialists, undergo surgery, and receive hospital care without having to pay privately for those services. Canadians are free to change doctors, change employers, and move to another part of the country without losing their public health insurance coverage. The *Canada Health Act* prohibits additional user fees or extra billing for services covered by public health insurance.

It is important to understand that the *Canada Health Act* privileges a model of health care that centres on physicians and hospitals. While public health insurance covers physician services and hospital care, it does not cover all health expenditures. Other services are funded privately, though there is some limited coverage through government programs targeted to seniors or low-income groups. To complicate matters, forms of privatization are affecting the scope of public—and private—health insurance in different provinces.

In *Exposing Privatization: Women and Health Care Reform in Canada*, Armstrong and colleagues (2002, 9) identify one form of privatization that is particularly germane to our discussion: privatizing the costs of health care by shifting the burden of payment to individuals. One strategy for accomplishing this is "delisting," which can be defined as a decrease in coverage for, and even the complete removal of, procedures, devices, and drugs from the list of "medically necessary" services that are publicly funded through provincial health insurance plans (see Ontario Health Coalition, 2003; Stabile & Ward, 2006). In Ontario, for instance, chiropractic, optometry, and community-based physical therapy services are among those that have been "delisted" (see Landry et al., 2006). Delisting has been associated with decreased use of services in some cases (Landry et al., 2006; Stabile & Ward, 2006); however, the gendered dimensions of this issue need to be examined more closely. When services are no longer covered by provincial public health insurance plans, they become the preserve of supplementary private health insurance plans or out-of-pocket payments.

At present no one source of information summarizes the number and characteristics of all Canadians who have private health insurance (Hurley & Guindon, 2008, 15). Data on various aspects of private health insurance indicate that a majority of Canadians hold some type of private coverage, with estimates suggesting that approximately 60 percent have some form of supplementary private health insurance for health services not covered by medicare (see Hurley & Guindon, 2008, for a discussion of different estimates). Supplementary insurance offers coverage for prescription drugs, dental care, eye care, physiotherapy, ambulance services, and many other health services. Many Canadians do not have private health insurance and must pay for these services directly out of pocket, if they can afford to do so.

Duplicate private health insurance provides coverage for the private delivery of services as an alternative to treatment in the public system. With duplicate health insurance, people may seek treatment from private health clinics in order to get faster access to care. This form of health insurance has not been part of the Canadian insurance market until recently. Several provinces have explicit legislation prohibiting the sale of duplicate health insurance for services already covered by medicare and requiring physicians to opt out of medicare if they choose to charge patients privately.

In recent years, owners of private clinics and patients seeking private treatment have challenged this legislation in the courts. In 2005, the Supreme Court of Canada ruled that Quebec's legislation banning duplicate private health insurance was in violation of the

*Quebec Charter of Human Rights and Freedoms* (*Chaoulli v. Quebec*). The court ruled that Quebec could not prohibit an individual from purchasing private health insurance and obtaining private care when faced with lengthy wait lists that delayed access to care in the public system. In response to the court's decision, the Quebec government initially worked on improving wait times in the public sector. However, the government also began to allow the purchase of duplicate private insurance coverage for three specific procedures that could be obtained from private surgical clinics. In 2009, the Quebec government further expanded the market for private insurance and private delivery of care by allowing private coverage for 56 different procedures and by allowing physicians to treat both medicare and privately financed patients. What is emerging is a parallel private system of care, in which those who can afford to pay privately are able to get faster access to treatment in private clinics (Picard, 2009).

Since 2005, the number of private clinics in Canada has grown and more people are paying privately for care outside the public system. Lawsuits have been launched in Alberta, Ontario, and British Columbia with the plaintiffs arguing that provincial restrictions on private insurance and extra billing limit access to private treatment and violate the *Canadian Charter of Rights and Freedoms* (Woodward, 2010).

Most Canadians strongly support the principle that health care is a basic right of citizenship, and that access to care should be based on need rather than ability to pay. An Ipsos Reid poll conducted in August 2010 found that only 11 percent of Canadians were in favour of more private payment for health care (Bauch, 2010). Despite the lack of public support, powerful groups continue to promote the privatization of health care financing through the expansion of private health insurance and the introduction of direct user fees for health services.

Proponents of these reforms argue that private insurance and direct user fees will inject additional money into the health care system, increase efficiency, discourage unnecessary use of health

services, and enable patients to get faster access to services purchased from private health clinics. Critics point out that privatization shifts the burden of payment to those who are sick, creates greater inequities in access to care, and increases health care
expenditures as more money goes into private profits and higher
administrative costs, while nothing is done to encourage a more
effective use of services (Bauch, 2010).

The way in which health care is financed determines who pays
for health care and the degree to which people are protected from
the financial risks of illness. Health care financing can influence
the availability of health services, access to care, the utilization of
services, and the resources available for providing care. It therefore has important consequences for those who need health services, those who provide health services, and those whose unpaid
care work is affected by gaps in services.

Other countries have adopted approaches to private health
insurance that differ from that used in Canada. Colombo and
Tapay (2004a) employ a typology that is useful for understanding
the different roles private health insurance can play. Where private health insurance is *primary*, it offers the only available access
to health insurance coverage for individuals who do not have
access to public health insurance, as in the US (Colombo & Tapay,
2004a, 31). As discussed above, *duplicate* private health insurance
provides those already covered under public health systems with
private coverage for the same services. Australia and Ireland offer
the most significant cases of duplicate insurance in the OECD
(Colombo & Tapay, 2004a, 34). *Complementary* private health
insurance is intended to complement publicly insured services or
those offered by other forms of private health insurance, covering
either all or part of costs not otherwise reimbursed, such as co-
payments. Both France and the US have significant complementary private health insurance markets (Colombo & Tapay, 2004a,
39). In contrast, as we have explained, the *supplementary* private
health insurance most common in Canada provides coverage for
health services that are not covered under public plans.

It is vital to understand that within different private health insurance markets, there are differences in the structure of benefits, premiums, and their method of calculation, cost-sharing arrangements, and insurers' relationships with health care providers (Colombo & Tapay, 2004a, 12). While all forms of private health insurance can be expected to have gendered implications due to women's particular roles as health care users, providers, and decision-makers, research on this topic that is published in English largely focuses on developments in the US.

## Gendered Inequities in Coverage

Access to private health insurance often varies according to gender. Men are more likely to have health insurance coverage through their own employment, while women are more likely to be insured as dependants through their spouses' insurance plans.

Aggregate statistics about insurance coverage hide important differences in the types of insurance coverage men and women have and the extent to which that coverage meets their health care needs (Miles & Parker, 1997). There is evidence of gender differences in forms of private insurance coverage in the European Union (Mossialos & Thomson, 2004), England (King & Mossialos, 2005), and Canada (Gibson & Fuller, 2006). However, as noted above, most of the research on gender and private health insurance comes from the United States, where private insurance is the only coverage available for most of the population.

Gender disparities in insurance coverage have been found in some studies of men and women experiencing illness. For example, a US study of women and men living with AIDS found that women were significantly less likely than men to have private health insurance (19.3 percent vs. 42.2 percent) (Bastian et al., 1993).

To understand gender disparities in private health insurance coverage, it is important to consider the main sources of private coverage: one's own employment, a spouse's employment, and individual purchase (Glied, Jack & Rachlin, 2008). Most private health insurance is available to people through employer-based group coverage offered as a part of workplace benefits. Male workers and women who are full-time workers with higher incomes tend to have higher rates of insurance coverage through employment (Salganicoff, Ranji & Wyn, 2005). According to Statistics Canada (2008), in 2005 less than half of female employees in Canada (46.7 percent) had employer-based health insurance benefits, compared to 56.2 percent of male employees.

Private health insurance coverage reflects patterns of gender segregation in the labour market (Dewar, 2000). Women are over-represented in low-paid, low-status occupations where they are less likely to receive health insurance benefits (Jecker, 1993; Miles & Parker, 1997; Brittle & Bird, 2007). They are more likely to work in small firms and in precarious or part-time jobs where private health insurance coverage is low or non-existent (Wyn et al., 2001). In Canada, women working in the service sector are in poorer health than women in other industries, and they also have the lowest rate of private insurance coverage (Cyrus & Curtis, 2004).

Linking health insurance to employment can create several problems for women. Anything that disrupts employment can lead to a loss of health insurance coverage. Women who lose their jobs or take time off work to raise children risk losing insurance coverage, as do women who leave work or cut back their hours in order to provide care for other family members. Women who work at home without pay are denied access to coverage unless they have a family member who can provide it (Jecker, 1993). Disruptions in coverage also make women more vulnerable to clauses in insurance policies that exclude or limit coverage for pre-existing conditions (Jecker, 1993; Miles & Parker, 1997).

When women do hold employment-based health insurance, this can affect their employment decisions. In the US, health insurance has been found to inhibit job mobility (Cooper & Monheit, 1993). Women facing illness may go to extraordinary lengths to obtain or retain employment in order to have health insurance. In a study of women with breast cancer, for instance, one-third of respondents stated "that they or their spouse stayed in a job to keep health insurance and implied that they wanted the freedom to leave" (Kinney et al., 1997, 186). Tying health care to employment is thus not only an exclusive practice, but one that can create particular challenges for those in need of care.

Although employment is the main avenue for private health insurance coverage for women in the US, employer-based health insurance has been in decline (Dewar, 2000; Glied, Jack & Rachlin, 2008). Gibson and Fuller (2006) point to a similar trend in Canada, finding supplementary health coverage fell by almost 25 percent between 1995 and 2000. As Wyn and colleagues (2001) explain, structural changes have led to the growth of jobs offering low pay and limited benefits. Meanwhile, increasing health care costs have led employers to cut health benefits, reduce coverage for families, and increase employees' share of premiums. Average deductibles in US employer-based plans tripled between 2000 and 2008 and quadrupled for employers with fewer than 200 employees (Kaiser Family Foundation, 2008 as cited in Rustgi, Doty & Collins, 2009). Workers are paying more for private health insurance, and often getting less.

Women have been especially hard hit by cutbacks in health insurance benefits. As Salganicoff, Ranji, and Wyn (2005, 47) explain, "higher premium costs, larger co-payments and increased cost-sharing combined with rapid growth in the cost of prescription drugs fall increasingly hard on women because of their higher use of health care services and their disproportionately lower incomes."

In the United States, coverage as a dependant is more prevalent among women than among men (Lambrew, 2001). Twenty-five percent of American women under 65 have private health insurance coverage through a spouse's employer (Kaiser Family Foundation, 2009). Significantly, this form of coverage is often available only to those in married heterosexual relationships. In the US, for instance, Claxton and colleagues (2009) found only 31 percent of firms reported offering health benefits to unmarried opposite-sex domestic partners, and only 21 percent reported offering health benefits to unmarried same-sex domestic partners.

As with coverage based on one's own employment, this indirect source of coverage has a variety of drawbacks. Dependants are susceptible to losing coverage when the primary policyholder loses his job or retires. They can also lose coverage when premium costs rise to unaffordable levels, or when employers reduce family coverage (Salganicoff, Ranji & Wyn, 2005; Kaiser Family Foundation, 2007). Since this source of coverage hinges on an individual's personal status, it can be lost in the event of divorce or the death of the primary policyholder (Salganicoff, Ranji & Wyn, 2005). Coverage as a dependant can also end when a young person reaches the maximum age limit for coverage under a parent's policy (Adams et al., 2007). Coverage tied to personal status can force women to make difficult choices. As Kinney and colleagues (1997) learned, some women have stayed in unsatisfactory marriages in order to retain insurance coverage to finance expensive cancer treatment.

Individually purchased health insurance plans are much less popular than employment-based group coverage. Lambrew (2001) suggests that those who purchase individual insurance coverage generally do so because they have few alternatives. In the United States, only 6 percent of women under 65 purchase individual health insurance coverage (Kaiser Family Foundation, 2009).

In the market for individual insurance coverage, commercial insurance companies use risk selection and risk rating as a way of lowering their costs and increasing their profits. In risk selection, private insurance companies routinely use sex, age, medical conditions, and other characteristics to estimate the health risks and potential health expenditures of their customers, and to determine eligibility for coverage. In risk rating, they use individual risk profiles to establish the level of premiums to be charged. These practices place women at a disadvantage, and they are particularly problematic for women with high health care needs.

Insurance companies expect women to make greater use of

health services, in part because of women's greater longevity and their reproductive health needs. Therefore, they tend to categorize women as "distinctly more expensive than males of the same age" (Ellis, 2008, 205). As the National Women's Law Center (2009, 3) has noted, insurance companies essentially treat women "like a pre-existing condition." By virtue of their sex, women are considered to have above-average risks and may face restrictions on their coverage or be charged higher premiums as a result. In much the same way, older people and those with pre-existing medical conditions may be charged more or denied coverage for some services (Mossialos & Thomson, 2004, 104; Davis et al., 2009, 15), placing women in these groups at an even greater disadvantage. It is not uncommon for insurance companies to exclude coverage for treatment of pre-existing conditions or to exclude coverage for maternity care. Due to risk selection, women who purchase individual health insurance in the US are healthier than women more generally (Lambrew, 2001). This reflects the difficulties encountered by women who are ill or have high health care needs, as well as the reality that women who have the lowest incomes often have the poorest health status (Salganicoff, Ranji & Wyn, 2005).

Sex-based risk profiles can result in dramatic gender gaps in premiums. The National Women's Law Center (2009) reports that women in some parts of the US pay up to 84 percent more than men for similar insurance coverage. While higher premiums are particularly a problem for women who purchase individual health insurance, they may also be found in group health insurance policies, where insurers are permitted to set premiums based on the number of women a business employs. There have been some efforts to reduce this inequity through regulation of the insurance industry. At the time of writing the practice of using sex when setting health insurance premiums has been prohibited in Australia (Colombo & Tapay, 2003), Ireland (Colombo & Tapay, 2004c), and some US states (National Women's Law Center, 2009), although we have little evidence of how effective this is in practice.

With employment, income, and personal status all liable to

change, the instability of private health insurance coverage is a key concern (Schoen, Duchon & Simantov, 1999; Salganicoff, Ranji & Wyn, 2005). Changes in one's personal circumstances can lead to loss of coverage for varying amounts of time. In the US, Salganicoff, Ranji, and Wyn (2005) found that 27 percent of women had been uninsured for part of the past year, and that one in five uninsured women lacked coverage for four years or more. Health conditions that develop during these gaps can later become classified as ineligible for coverage (Salganicoff, Ranji & Wyn, 2005), effectively denying coverage when the need for such coverage is greatest.

In the US, the cost of health care poses a significant problem even for women who have private insurance (Kinney et al., 1997, 183; Almeida, Dubay & Ko, 2001; Salganicoff, Ranji & Wyn, 2005; Rustgi, Doty & Collins, 2009). A study of breast cancer patients found that even women with comprehensive health insurance had high treatment costs, with the majority of out-of-pocket expenses arising from co-payments for hospitalization and physician services (Arozullah et al., 2004).

Women as a group face serious challenges in obtaining and maintaining private health insurance coverage, and different groups of women are particularly disadvantaged in this regard. Private health insurance coverage is influenced by many factors, including age, gender, income, race, employment status, level of education, and location. In the US, a women's health survey found that 89 percent of women from higher income families have private health insurance coverage, compared with 75 percent of women from modest income households, 49 percent of women in "near poor" households, and only 24 percent of women in poor households. Seventy-six percent of White women have private health insurance compared with 62 percent of African-American women and only 42 percent of Latina women. Women who are employed full-time have higher rates of coverage than women who are employed part-time, self-employed, or not employed. Women who are married have higher rates of coverage than women who are living with unmarried partners, or who are divorced, separated, or widowed. Women with private health insurance tend to have higher levels of education and better health than women without private insurance (Salganicoff, Ranji & Wyn, 2005).

There is evidence to suggest that women with serious mental illness and women with histories of abuse are more likely to rely on public rather than private health insurance (Belcher et al., 1995; Evins & Chescheir, 1996). Bogarin (2005) found that women with histories of domestic violence are often unable to obtain private health insurance because insurance companies consider them to be too high risk. Corliss (2004) found that women and men in same-sex and opposite-sex unmarried partnerships are less likely than married couples to have private health insurance, but particularly less likely to have coverage through employer-based health benefits. A study of private health insurance in the European Union found that those who purchase supplementary health insurance tend to come from higher income groups, have higher occupational status, and live in wealthier regions (Mossialos & Thomson, 2004).

Overall, disparities in private health insurance coverage reflect the broader patterns of inequality found within social relations based on gender, class, race, age, ability, health status, and other forms of difference.

# Gendered Inequities in Care

Inequities in private health insurance coverage have different consequences, depending on the role that private health insurance plays in health care financing. In Canada, where private insurance provides supplementary coverage for services not covered by medicare, the lack of private insurance can mean limited access to prescription drugs, dental care, eye care, and numerous other health services. In the US there is no universal public health insurance, and most people have to rely on private health insurance as their primary protection against the costs of illness. In this context, a lack of private health insurance coverage can be deadly. In 2006, an estimated 22,000 people in the US died unnecessarily because they did not have health insurance (Dorn, 2008).

Lack of health insurance increases the risk of death and disease, as well as the risk of financial hardship. It can profoundly affect access to care and quality of life. Those without insurance may forego or delay treatment, often leading to more serious health problems. Inability to pay for health care services can lead to untreated morbidity, reduced access to care, long-term impoverishment, and irrational use of drugs (Ostlin, 2005). Lack of insurance to pay for formal care providers can lead to a greater burden of care work for unpaid caregivers, most of whom are women (Forget et al., 2005, 126).

Over 17 million women in the United States have no public or private health insurance coverage (Kaiser Family Foundation, 2009). According to the 2008 Kaiser Women's Health Survey, among uninsured women aged 18 to 64, 56 percent reported that they did not get needed care because of the cost, 53 percent reported that they had no regular doctor, 34 percent reported that they did not fill prescriptions because of cost, and 34 percent did not get a Pap test (Kaiser Family Foundation, 2009). "Uninsured women are more likely to lack adequate access to care, get a lower standard of care when they are in the health system, and have poorer health outcomes" (Kaiser Family Foundation, 2009). Uninsured women are much less likely to use health services than women with either public or private health insurance (Taylor, Larson & Correa-de-Araujo, 2006).

A number of research studies in the US have looked at specific health services and compared the treatment of privately insured women with the treatment of those who are uninsured or covered by public insurance. For example, Coburn and colleagues (2008) found that breast cancer patients with private health insurance presented with lower stage cancer were more likely to receive surgical treatment, more likely to have breast

conservation surgery, and more likely to have breast recon-
struction following mastectomy than women with public or no
insurance. Battaglia and colleagues (2007) and Ferrante and colleagues (2007) found that privately insured patients had more
timely follow-up to abnormal breast cancer screening. There is
some evidence to suggest that privately insured women have
higher rates of Pap testing (Cherry et al., 2008), greater access to
prenatal care (Braveman et al., 1993), and higher rates of mammography (David et al., 2005; Cohen et al., 1997). Culwell and
Feinglass (2007b) found that privately insured women were
much more likely to use prescription contraceptives, while Borrero and colleagues (2007) found that they were less likely to
undergo tubal sterilizations. A study of HIV-positive women
found that those with private insurance were much more likely
to report use of highly active antiretroviral therapy, "suggesting that women without private health insurance coverage may
have reduced access to the most effective treatments for HIV"
(Cook et al., 2002, 86). Women with private insurance are more
likely to use infertility services, particularly medications that
induce ovulation, but they are not more likely to use assisted
reproductive technology, since it is typically not covered by private health insurance policies (Farley & Webb, 2007). In Canada,
a study of women with breast cancer found that patients with
private health insurance were more likely to use complementary
and alternative medicine (Grey et al., 2003). In Australia, Korda
and colleagues (2009) found that inequalities in the use of dental
and allied health services are partly explained by inequalities in
private insurance coverage. While it is hard to generalize from
these studies in terms of particular treatments, they do indicate
that private health insurance creates inequities in care between
those who are privately insured and those who are not.

For many women who are underinsured, private health insurance does not provide adequate protection, the costs of care
become a financial burden, and their access to care is compromised. Research suggests that underinsurance has gendered

consequences, with women facing greater financial barriers to care. Rustgi, Doty, and Collins (2009) found that nearly 70 percent of underinsured women reported cost-related problems in getting needed care, compared with about half of underinsured men. Women who were underinsured reported financial barriers to care nearly as often as women who were uninsured. One US study found that 19 percent of women with private health insurance spent $100 or more per month on medications, and 13 percent didn't take their medications or took less than the prescribed dose (Salganicoff, Ranji & Wyn, 2005).

By excluding pre-existing conditions or particular health services, placing limits on benefits, and requiring pre-approval of treatments, some private insurance policies fail to provide coverage for the conditions women have or the treatments they seek. Salganicoff, Ranji, and Wyn (2005) found that 16 percent of insured women in the US had been denied approval or payment for a health care service, and 11 percent were not able to see a specialist when they thought one was needed.

Private health insurance offers limited coverage for mental health services. Those with mental health problems may face higher premiums, higher co-payments, and restrictions on services (Barry et al., 2003). Women seeking treatment can find benefit limits leave them with inadequate protection for their mental health care needs (Jenkins, 2009). This is particularly relevant for Canada, given the limited services available through the public system.

Private health insurance policies vary in the levels of protection they offer and the range of services they cover; they may not provide coverage for the full range of women's health needs. There are inconsistencies in coverage for maternity care, abortions, and other sexual and reproductive health services (Kurth et al., 2001; Culwell & Feinglass, 2007a). There has been some effort to address these problems through regulation of the private insurance industry. Some jurisdictions have required private insurers to cover a range of health services specific to women, including mammography, cervical cancer screening, contraceptives, and reproductive health services (Kaiser Family Foundation, 2003). Some effort has also been made to regulate adequate coverage for mental health services (Barry et al., 2003).

While the research shows that private health insurance improves women's access to services covered by their insurance, this does not necessarily mean the best care. Private insurance coverage may encourage the overuse of some health services, particularly when there are financial incentives to do so. Colbert and colleagues (2004) found that women with private insurance began receiving mammograms earlier than those without private insurance. This may or may not be a good thing. A significant body of research shows an association between private insurance coverage and use of Caesarean section in countries, including Australia (Fisher, Smith & Astbury, 1995; Shorten & Shorten, 2004), Chile (Murray, 2000; Murray & Pradenas, 1997), Greece (Mossialos et al., 2005a; Mossialos et al., 2005b), and the US (Gilbert, 1990, 1991; Hangsleben et al., 1995; Woolbright, 1996). Higher Caesarean section rates for the privately insured have been linked to financial and convenience incentives created for physicians (Mossialos et al., 2005a; Murray & Elston, 2005). Murray and Elston (2005) interviewed obstetricians to gain insight into the causes of higher Caesarean section rates in the private sector in Chile, and found participants often regulated the timing of births in order to manage their own time — and earning capacity — most efficiently. Such findings suggest the role of financial gain in promoting this procedure among privately insured women, a factor that other research on private health insurance would do well to consider.

Further privatization of health care financing through the introduction of user fees or the expansion of private health insurance poses the risk of increasing inequities in access to care. In 2005, the European office of the World Health Organization (WHO) published a report that examined the impact of four types of health reforms on gender equity. In reviewing the international evidence on health care financing, the report concluded that "There is substantial evidence from both high-income and low-income countries that taxes and social insurance schemes provide the most equitable basis for health financing. Other schemes, such as private insurance or direct out-of-pocket payment, are likely to increase inequities, particularly in access to care and health-seeking behaviour and this may affect women more, as they generally have fewer financial resources" (Ostlin, 2005, 12).

Proponents of private health insurance argue that it provides patients with more timely access to care, but the evidence does not support this claim unless one considers only the experience of those who purchase treatment in private clinics. Duplicate private health insurance and the growth of private health facilities in Australia have not reduced wait times for treatment in the public system (Hurley et al., 2002). While those with private insurance are frequently able to purchase more timely access to care in private clinics, the growth of private insurance and private clinics can create longer waiting lists for those seeking treatment in the public system (Canadian Health Services Research Foundation, 2005). A study of health financing arrangements in five different countries found "no grounds for believing that the existence of a privately insured sector parallel to the public sector reduces overall waiting lists or times" (Tuohy, Flood & Stabile, 2004, 376). In fact, this study found that expansion of private insurance and the growth of a parallel private system of care led to longer waits for care in the public system.

When private insurance pays health care providers at higher rates, there is a disincentive for physicians to treat publicly insured patients. Doctors and other health care personnel may be drawn away from the public system, leaving it understaffed and less able to provide timely access to care. This could create staff shortages in the public system that would lengthen wait times and make care less accessible to those without private insurance.

Women rely more heavily than men on public health care, in part because of their greater health care needs, but also because they have lower incomes, and are less likely to be covered by forms of private health insurance (Forget et al., 2005; Gómez Gómez, 2000).

Expansion of private health insurance promotes the growth of a parallel system of private care. The growth of a parallel private system threatens to undermine the public health care systems on which women disproportionately depend. Privatization may lead women to experience greater barriers to accessing and providing care as patients waiting for care in the public system, as unpaid care providers, and as public health care workers coping with staff shortages.

According to the World Health Organization, an expansion of private health insurance can undermine public support for financing public health care (WHO, 2006). Where individuals with private insurance are entitled to opt out of public health insurance, the state's capacity for pooling risk is reduced, threatening the long-term financial stability of public health care systems (Thomson & Mossialos, 2004). In Chile, where individuals enrol in either public or private health insurance, Sapelli and Torche (2001) found that private insurers maximized profits through risk selection, leaving the public system to finance care for those with the greatest health care needs. When private coverage is publicly subsidized, this results in additional public expense. Hurley and colleagues (2002, 19) describe Australia's policy of subsidizing private insurance as "a dramatic failure that, on balance, annually costs the public purse billions of dollars." Thomson and Mossialos (2004, 4) caution that tax subsidies for private health insurance are inefficient, distort signals about the real price of insurance, and generate transaction costs. Nor do public subsidies for private health insurance affect women and men equally. Efforts to subsidize private health insurance through a system of tax credits are not enough to make this form of insurance available, affordable, or sufficient for women (Collins, Berkson & Downey, 2002).

Some researchers contend that better regulation can help to improve the functioning of private health insurance and limit its negative impact on public systems (Thomson & Mossialos, 2004; Greb, 2005; Colombo & Tapay, 2004b). However, as Hurley and colleagues (2002) warn, experience shows it is extremely challenging to regulate health insurance companies to pursue public objectives. In theory as well as practice, the goal of health care for those in need is difficult to reconcile with the pursuit of profit by private insurers.

# References

Adams, S.H., Newacheck, P.W., Park, M.J., Brindis, C.D. & Irwin, C.E., Jr. (2007). Health insurance across vulnerable ages: Patterns and disparities from adolescence to the early 30s. *Pediatrics 119*(5), e1033–e1039.

Almeida, R.A., Dubay, L.C. & Ko, G. (2001). Access to care and use of health services by low-income women. *Health Care Financing Review 22*(4), 27–47.

Angel, R., Lein, L. & Henrici, J. (2006). *Poor families in America's health care crisis*. Cambridge: Cambridge University Press.

Angus, L.D.G., Cottam, D.R., Gorecki, P.J., Mourello, R., Ortega, R.E. & Adamski, J. (2003). DRG, costs, and reimbursement following roux-en-Y gastric bypass: An economic appraisal. *Obesity Surgery 13*, 591–595.

Armstrong, P., Amaratunga, C., Bernier, J., Grant, K., Pederson, A. & Willson, K. (Eds.). (2002). *Exposing privatization: Women and health care reform in Canada*. Aurora: Garamond Press.

Arozullah, A.M., Calhoun, E.A., Wolf, M., Finley, D.K., Fitzner, K.A., Heckinger, E.A., et al. (2004). The financial burden of cancer: Estimates from a study of insured women with breast cancer. *Journal of Supportive Oncology 2*(3), 271–278.

Ayanian, J.Z., Kohler, B.A., Abe, T. & Epstein, A.M. (1993). The relation between health insurance coverage and clinical outcomes among women with breast cancer. *New England Journal of Medicine 329*(5), 326–331.

Barry, C.L., Gabel, J.R., Frank, R.G., Hawkins, S., Whitmore, H.H. & Pickreign, J.D. (2003). Design of mental health benefits: Still unequal after all these years. *Health Affairs 22*(5), 127–137.

Bastian, L., Bennett, C.L., Adams, J., Waskin, H., Divine, G. & Edlin, B.R. (1993). Differences between men and women with HIV-related pneumocystis carinii pneumonia: Experience from 3,070 cases in New York City in 1987. *Journal of Acquired Immune Deficiency Syndromes 6*(6), 617–623.

Battaglia, T.A., Roloff, K., Posner, M.A. & Freund, K.M. (2007). Improving follow-up to abnormal breast cancer screening in an urban population: A patient navigation intervention. *Cancer 109*(2 Supplement), 359–367.

Bauch, H. (2010). Funding crunch: Prescriptions for health care diverge sharply. *Montreal Gazette*, October 30. Retrieved from http://www.montrealgazette.com/health/Funding+crunch+Prescriptions+health+care+diverge+sharply/3750135/story.html

Belcher, J.R., DeForge, B.R., Thompson, J.W. & Myers, C.P. (1995). Psychiatric hospital care and changes in insurance coverage strategies: A national study. *The Journal of Mental Health Administration 22*(4), 377–387.

Bogarin, S.A. (2005). *The perceptions of female survivors of intimate partner violence who lack healthcare coverage.* M.S.W. thesis, California State University, Long Beach. Publication no.: AAT1429222. Proquest Dissertations and Theses 2005. Section 6080, Part 0452, 87 pages.

Borrell, C., Fernandez, E., Schiaffino, A., Benach, J., Rajmil, L., Villalbi, J.R. & Segura, A. (2001). Social class inequalities in the use of and access to health services in Catalonia, Spain: What is the influence of supplemental private health insurance? *International Journal for Quality in Health Care 13*(2): 117–125.

Borrero, S., Schwarz, E.B., Reeves, M.F., Bost, J.E., Creinin, M.D. & Ibrahim, S.A. (2007). Race, insurance status, and tubal sterilization. *Obstetrics & Gynecology 109*(1), 94–100.

Braveman, P., Bennett, T., Lewis, C., Egerter, S. & Showstack, J. (1993). Access to prenatal care following major Medicaid eligibility expansions. *Journal of the American Medical Association 269*(10), 1285–1289.

Brittle, C. & Bird, C.E. (2007). *Literature review on effective sex- and gender-based systems/models of care.* Office on Women's Health, US Department of Health and Human Services. Retrieved from http://www.4women.gov/owh/multidisciplinary/ reports/GenderBasedMedicine/FinalOWHReport.pdf

Canada Health Act, R.S.C. 1985, c. C-6.

Canadian Health Services Research Foundation. (2005). *Myth: A parallel private system would reduce waiting times in the public system.* Retrieved from http://www.chsrf.ca/mythbusters/html/myth17_e. php#viii

Canadian Institute for Health Information. (2010). *National health expenditure trends, 1975 to 2010.* Ottawa: Canadian Institute for Health Information.

Case, B.G.S., Himmelstein, D.U. & Woolhandler, S. (2002). No care for the caregivers: Declining health insurance coverage for health care personnel and their children, 1988–1998. *American Journal of Public Health 92*(3), 404–408.

Cherry, D.K., Hing, E., Woodwell, D.A. & Rechtsteiner, E.A. (2008). National ambulatory medical care survey: 2006 summary. *National Health Statistics Reports 3*(August 6), 1–40.

Claxton, G., DiJulio, B., Finder, B., Lundy, J., McHugh, M., Osei-Anto, A., et al. (2009). *Employer health benefits 2009.* Menlo Park and Chicago: The Henry J. Kaiser Family Foundation and Health Research and Educational Trust.

Coburn, N., Fulton, J., Pearlman, D.N., Law, C., DiPaolo, B. & Cady, B. (2008). Treatment variation by insurance status for breast cancer patients. *The Breast Journal 14*(2), 128–134.

Cohen, R.A., Bloom, B., Simpson, G. & Parsons, P.E. (1997). Access to health care. Part 3: Older adults. *Vital and Health Statistics,* Series 10. Data from the National Health Survey, 198, 1–32.

Colbert, J.A., Kaine, E.M., Bigby, J., Smith, D.N., Moore, R.H., Rafferty, E., et al. (2004). The age at which women begin mammographic screening. *Cancer 101*(8), 1850–1859.

Collins, S.R., Berkson, S.B. & Downey, D.A. (2002). *Health insurance tax credits: Will they work for women?* The Commonwealth Fund. Retrieved from http://www.commonwealthfund.org/~/media/ Files/Publications/Fund%20Report/2003/Jan/Health%20Insurance%20Tax%20Credits%20%20Will%20They%20Work%20 for%20Women/collins_creditswomen_589%20pdf.pdf

Colombo, F. & Tapay, N. (2003). *Private health insurance in Australia: A case study.* OECD Health Working Papers no.8. Paris: OECD.

Colombo, F. & Tapay, N. (2004a). *Private health insurance in OECD countries*. OECD Health Project. Paris: OECD.

Colombo, F. & Tapay, N. (2004b). *Private health insurance in OECD countries: The benefits and costs for individuals and health systems*. OECD Health Working Papers no. 15. Retrieved from http://ideas.repec.org/p/oec/elsaad/15-en.html

Colombo, F. & Tapay, N. (2004c). *Private health insurance in Ireland: A case study*. OECD Health Working Papers no. 10. Paris: OECD.

Cook, J.A., Cohen, M.H., Grey, D., Kirstein, L., Burke, J., Anastos, K., et al. (2002). Use of highly active antiretroviral therapy in a cohort of HIV-seropositive women. *American Journal of Public Health 92*(1), 82–87.

Cooper, P.F. & Monheit, A.C. (1993). Does employment-related health insurance inhibit job mobility? *Inquiry 30*(4), 400–416.

Corliss, H.L. (2004). *An examination of the role of sexual orientation in generating disparities in health and health care*. Ph.D. dissertation, University of California, Los Angeles. Publication no.: AAT 3155001. Proquest Dissertations and Theses 2004. Section 0031, Part 0573, 236 pages.

Culwell, K.R. & Feinglass, J. (2007a). The association of health insurance with use of prescription contraceptives. *Perspectives on Sexual and Reproductive Health 39*(4), 226–230.

Culwell, K.R. & Feinglass, J. (2007b). Changes in prescription contraceptive use, 1995–2002: The effect of insurance status. *Obstetrics & Gynecology 110*(6), 1371–1378.

Cyrus, T.L. & Curtis, L.J. (2004). *Trade agreements, the health-care sector, and women's health*. Status of Women Canada. Retrieved from http://www.swccfc.gc.ca/pubs/pubspr/0662374215/200408_066237 4215_e.pdf

David, M.M., Ko, L., Prudent, N., Green, E.H., Posner, M.A. & Freund, K.M. (2005). Mammography use. *Journal of the National Medical Association 97*(2), 253–261.

Davis, K., Stremikis, K., Schoen C., Collins, S.R., Doty, M.M., Rustgi, S.D., & Nicholson, J.L. (2009). *Front and center: Ensuring that health reform puts people first*. The Commonwealth Fund. Retrieved from http://www.commonwealthfund.org/~/media /Files/Publications/

Fund%20Report/2009/Jun/Front%20and%20Center/1280_Davis_
front_and_center_FINAL_06022009.pdf

Dewar, D.M. (2000). Gender impacts on health insurance coverage:
Findings for unmarried full-time employees. *Women's Health Issues*
10, 268–277.

Dorn, S. (2008). Uninsured and dying because of it: Updating the Institute of Medicine analysis on the impact of uninsurance on mortality. Urban Institute. Retrieved from http://www.urban.org/
UploadedPDF/411588_uninsured_dying.pdf

Dorn, S., Alteras, T. & Meyer, J.A. (2005). Early implementation of the
health coverage tax credit in Maryland, Michigan, and North Carolina: A case study summary. The Commonwealth Fund. Publication no. 806. Retrieved from http://www.commonwealthfund.org/
usr_doc/806_dorn_earlyimplementationhct.pdf

Dubay, L. (1999). *Expansions in public health insurance and crowd out: What
the evidence says*. Issue Paper. The Kaiser Project on Incremental
Health Reform. The Henry J. Kaiser Family Foundation. Retrieved
from http://www.kff.org/uninsured/loadercfm?url=/commonspot/
security/getfile.cfm&PageID=13305

Ellis, R.P. (2008). Risk adjustment in health care markets: Concepts and
applications. In M. Lu & E. Jonsson (Eds.), *Financing health care:
New ideas for a changing society* (pp. 177–222). Weinheim: Wiley.

Evins, G. & Chescheir, N. (1996). Prevalence of domestic violence
among women seeking abortion services. *Women's Health Issues*
6(4), 204–210.

Farley, O.S. & Webb, N.J. (2007). Utilization of infertility services: How
much does money matter? *Health Services Research* 42(3), 971–989.

Ferrante, J.M., Rovi, S., Das, K. & Kim, S. (2007). Family physicians
expedite diagnosis of breast disease in urban minority women.
*Journal of the American Board of Family Medicine* 20(1), 52–59.

Fisher, J., Smith, A. & Astbury, J. (1995). Private health-insurance and
a healthy personality—new risk-factors for obstetric intervention.
*Journal of Psychosomatic Obstetrics and Gynecology* 16(1), 1–9.

Flood, C.M., Stabile, M. & Kontic, S. (2005). Finding health policy "arbi-
trary": The evidence on waiting, dying, and two-tiered systems.
In C.M. Flood, K. Roach & S. Lorne (Eds.), *Access to care, access to*

*justice: The legal debate over private health insurance in Canada.* Pp. 296–320. Toronto: University of Toronto Press.

Forget, E.L., Deber, R., Roos, L. & Walld, R. (2005). Canadian health reform: A gender analysis. *Feminist Economics 11*, 123–141.

Gibson, D. & Fuller, C. (2006). *The bottom line: The truth behind private health insurance in Canada.* Edmonton: Parkland Institute.

Gilbert, E. (1990). Unnecessary C-sections hit patients. *National Underwriter 94*(4), 16.

Gilbert, E. (1991). Some hospitals found to cash-in on C-sections. *National Underwriter 95*(5), 6.

Glied, S., Jack, K. & Rachlin, J. (2008). Women's health insurance coverage 1980–2005. *Women's Health Issues 18*(1), 7–16.

Gómez Gómez, E. (2000). *Equity, gender, and health policy reform in Latin America and the Caribbean.* Washington: Pan American Health Organization.

Greb, S. (2005). The role of private health insurance in social health insurance countries—implications for Canada. In C.M. Flood, K. Roach & S. Lorne (Eds.), *Access to care, access to justice: The legal debate over private health insurance in Canada*.pp. 278–295. Toronto: University of Toronto Press.

Grey, R.E., Fitch, M., Goel, V., Franssen, E. & Labrecque, M. (2003). Utilization of complementary/alternative services by women with breast cancer. *Journal of Health & Social Policy 16*(4), 75–84.

Hangsleben, K., Jones, M., Liahoagberg, B., Skovholt, C. & Wingeier, R. (1995). Medicaid and non-medicaid prenatal care by nurse-midwives. *Journal of Nurse-Midwifery 40*(4), 320–327.

Hurley, J., et al. 2002. *Parallel private health insurance in Australia: A cautionary tale and lessons for Canada.* Discussion Paper 448, Centre for Economic Policy Research, Research School of Social Sciences, Australian National University. Retrieved from http://www.canadiandoctorsformedicare.ca/Australia Hurley ParallelPrivateHealthInsuranceinAustralia.pdf

Hurley, J. & Guindon, G.E. (2008). *Private health insurance in Canada.* CHEPA Working Paper Series Paper 08-04. This paper is forthcoming as a chapter in S. Thomson, E. Mossialos & R.G. Evans (Eds.), *Private health insurance and medical savings accounts: Lessons from international experience*. London: Cambridge University Press.

Institute of Medicine (US). Committee on Redesigning Health Insurance Performance Measures, Payment, and Performance Improvement Programs. (2006). *Performance measurement: Accelerating improvement*. Washington: National Academies Press.

Jecker, N. (1993). Can an employer-based health-insurance system be just? *Journal of Health Politics, Policy, and Law 18*(3), 657–673.

Jenkins, A. (2007). *Women and private health insurance: A review of the issues*. Report Commissioned by Women and Health Care Reform. http://www.womenandhealthcarereform.ca/en/work_insurance.html.

Jenkins, A. (2009). Falling through the cracks: Women, depression, and health insurance coverage in Ontario. M.A. thesis, York University, Toronto. Masters Abstracts International, 47(04), Publication number: AAT MR45948. Proquest Dissertations and Theses, 144 pages.

Kaiser Family Foundation. (2003). *Women's access to care: A state level analysis of key health policies*. No. 3326. Menlo Park: The Henry J. Kaiser Family Foundation.

Kaiser Family Foundation. (2007). *Women's health insurance coverage*. Retrieved from http://www.kff.org/womenshealth/upload/6000_05.pdf

Kaiser Family Foundation. (2008a). *Health care and the 2008 elections: Women's health policy*. Retrieved fromhttp://www.kff.org/womenshealth/upload /7822.pdf

Kaiser Family Foundation. (2008b). *Abortion in the US: Utilization, financing, and access*. Menlo Park: The Henry J. Kaiser Family Foundation.

Kaiser Family Foundation. (2009). *Women's health insurance coverage*. Retrieved from http://www.kff.org/womenshealth/upload/6000-08.pdf

King, D. & Mossialos, E. (2005). The determinants of private medical insurance prevalence in England, 1997–2000. *Health Services Research 40*(1), 195–212.

Kinney, E.D., Freund, D.A., Camp, M.E., Jordan, K.A. & Mayfield, M.C. (1997). Serious illness and private health coverage: A unique problem calling for unique solutions. *The Journal of Law, Medicine &*

*Ethics 25*(2–3), 180–191.

Korda, R.J., Banks, E., Clements, M.S. & Young, A.F. (2009). Is inequity undermining Australia's "universal" health care system? Socio-economic inequalities in the use of specialist medical and non-medical ambulatory health care. *Australian and New Zealand Journal of Public Health 33*(5), 458.

Kurth, A., Bielinski, L., Graap, K., Conniff, J. & Connell, F. (2001). Reproductive and sexual health benefits in private health insurance plans in Washington State. *Family Planning Perspectives 33*(4), 153–160 and 179.

Lambrew, J.M. (2001). *Diagnosing disparities in health insurance for women: A prescription for change.* The Commonwealth Fund. Retrieved from http://www.cmwf.org/usr_doc/lambrew_disparities_493.pdf

Landry, M.D., et al. (2006). Assessing the consequences of delisting publicly funded community-based physical therapy on self-reported health in Ontario, Canada: A prospective cohort study. *Journal of Rehabilitation Research 29*(4), 303–307.

Merzel, C. (2000). Gender differences in health care access indicators in an urban, low-income community. *American Journal of Public Health 90*, 909–916.

Miles, S. & Parker, K. (1997). Men, women, and health insurance. *New England Journal of Medicine 336*, 218–221.

Monheit, A.C., Vistnes, J.P. & Eisenberg, J.M. (2001). Moving to medicare: Trends in the health insurance status of near-elderly workers, 1987–1996. *Health Affairs 20*(2), 204–213.

Mossialos, E.S., Allin, K., Karras, K. & Davaki, K. (2005a). An investigation of Caesarean sections in three Greek hospitals: The impact of financial incentives and convenience. *European Journal of Public Health 15*, 288–295.

Mossialos, E., Costa-Font, J., Davaki, K. & Karras, K. (2005b). Is there "patient selection" in the demand for private maternity care in Greece? *Applied Economics Letters 12*(1), 7–12.

Mossialos, E. & Thomson, S. (2004). *Voluntary health insurance in the European Union.* Brussels: World Health Organization on behalf of the European Observatory on Health Systems and Policies. Retrieved from http://www.euro.who.int/ Document/ E84885.pdf

Murray, S.F. (2000). Relation between private health insurance and high rates of Caesarean section in Chile: Qualitative and quantitative study. *British Medical Journal 321*(7275), 1501–1505.

Murray, S. & Elston, M. (2005). The promotion of private health insurance and its implications for the social organisation of healthcare: A case study of private sector obstetric practice in Chile. *Sociology of Health & Illness 27*(6), 701–721.

Murray, S. & Pradenas, F. (1997). Cesarean birth trends in Chile, 1986 to 1994. *Birth: Issues in Perinatal Care 24*(4), 258–263.

National Women's Law Center. (2008). *Nowhere to turn: How the individual health insurance market fails women*. Retrieved from http://action.nwlc.org/site/PageServer?pagename=nowheretoturn

National Women's Law Center. (2009). *Still nowhere to turn: Insurance companies treat women like a pre-existing condition*. Retrieved from http://www.nwlc.org/pdf/stillnowheretoturn.pdf

O'Rand, A.M. & Henretta, J.C. (1999). *Labor markets and occupational welfare in the United States. Age and inequality: Diverse pathways through later life*. Boulder: Westview Press.

Ontario Health Coalition. (2003). *Privatization of medicare and women*. Retrieved from http://www.web.net/~ohc/docs/fact_sheet-priv.htm

Ostlin, P. (2005). *What is the evidence about the effects of health care reforms on gender equity, particularly in health?* Health Evidence Network Report. Copenhagen: World Health Organization Regional Office for Europe. Retrieved from www.euro.who.int/__data/assets/pdf_file/0015/73230/E87674.pdf

Picard, A. (2009). Private health care slips under radar. *Globe and Mail*, July 16. Retrieved from http://www.theglobeandmail.com/life/health/private-health-care-slips-under-radar/article1220145/

Rhine, S.L.W. & Chu Ng, Y.C. (1998). The effect of employment status on private health insurance coverage: 1977 and 1987. *Health Economics 7*(1), 63–79.

Rustgi, S.D., Doty, M.M. & Collins, S.R. (2009). *Women at risk: Why many women are forgoing needed health care*. Issue Brief. The Commonwealth Fund. Retrieved from http://thecommonwealthfund.net/~/media/Files/Publications/Issue%20Brief/2009/May/Women%20

at%20Risk/PDF_1262_Rustgi_women_at_risk_issue_brief_Final.
pdf

Salganicoff, A., Ranji, U.R. & Wyn, R. (2005). *Women and health care: A national profile.* Henry J. Kaiser Family Foundation. Retrieved from http://www.kff.org/womenshealth/upload/Women-and-Health-Care-ANational-Profile-Key-Findings-from-the-Kaiser-Women-s-Health-Survey.pdf

Sapelli, C. & Torche, A. (2001). The mandatory health insurance system in Chile: Explaining the choice between public and private insurance. *International Journal of Health Care Finance and Economics 1*(2), 97.

Schoen, C., Duchon, L. & Simantov, E. (1999). The link between health and economic security for working age women. Issue Brief. The Commonwealth Fund. Retrieved from: http://www.commonwealthfund.org/~/media/Files/Publications/Issue%20Brief/1999/May/The%20Link%20Between%20Health%20and%20Economic%20Security%20for%20Working%20Age%20Women/healtheconomic_brief%20pdf.pdf

Shorten, B. & Shorten, A. (2004). Impact of private health insurance incentives on obstetric outcomes in NSW hospitals. *Australian Health Review 27*, 27–38.

Stabile, M. & Ward, C. (2006). The effects of delisting publicly funded health care services. In C.M. Beach, R.P. Chaykowski, S. Shortt, F. St-Hilaire &A. Sweetman (Eds.), *Health services restructuring in Canada: New evidence and new directions* (pp. 83–110). Kingston: McGill-Queen's University Press.

Statistics Canada. (2008). *Workplace and employee survey compendium 2005.* Section 4 Compensation practices, Table 4.4 Employee's non-wage benefits, 2005, p. 50 (Catalogue no. 71-585-X). Retrieved from http://www.statcan.gc.ca/pub/71-585-x/2008001/table/table4p4-eng.htm

Taylor, A.K., Larson, S. & Correa-de-Araujo, R. (2006). Women's health care utilization and expenditures. *Women's Health Issues 16*(2), 66–79.

Thomson, S. & Mossialos, E. (2004). *What are the equity, efficiency, cost containment, and choice implications of private health care funding in western Europe?* Health Evidence Network Report. Copenhagen:

World Health Organization Regional Office for Europe. Retrieved from http://www.euro.who.int/Document/E83334.pdf

Tuohy, C.H., Flood, C.M. & Stabile, M. (2004). How does private finance affect public health systems? Marshalling evidence from the OECD. *Journal of Health Politics, Policy, and Law 29*, 359–396.

Woodward, C. (2010). Legal challenges may imperil medicare, public health care advocates say. *Canadian Medical Association Journal* (November 11). Retrieved from http://www.cmaj.ca/earlyreleases/11nov10-legal-challenges-may-imperil-medicare-public-health-care-advocates-say.pdf

Woolbright, L. (1996). Why is the cesarean delivery rate so high in Alabama? An examination of risk factors, 1991–1993. *Birth: Issues in Perinatal Care 23*(1), 20–25.

World Health Organization (WHO). (2005). *The health systems responsiveness analytical guidelines for surveys in the multi-country survey study.* Geneva: World Health Organization.

World Health Organization (WHO). (2006). *Health financing: A basic guide.* Geneva: World Health Organization.

Wyn, R., Solís, B., Ojeda, V.D. & Pourat, N. (2001). *Falling through the cracks: Health insurance coverage of low income women.* Menlo Park: The Henry J. Kaiser Family Foundation.

Zimmerman, M.K. & Hill, S.A. (2006). Health care as a gendered system. In J. Saltzman Chafetz (Ed.), *Handbook of sociology of gender* (pp. 483–518). New York: Springer.

CHAPTER 11

# Overweight, Obesity, and Health Care

KAREN R. GRANT

At the start of 2011, the CBC launched a multi-faceted set of programs on television, radio, and online tackling Canada's national weight problem. *Live Right Now* profiles Canadians' sedentary ways and their less than healthy eating habits, and provides expert advice and programs on making small changes in diet and exercise, aiming to have a major impact on Canadians' weight and health. In addition to tracking a select group of Canadians trying to live healthier lifestyles, the CBC is encouraging Canadians to take the "Million Pound Challenge" (modelled after the Canadian government's 2004 "One Tonne Challenge" to reduce greenhouse emissions). One month into the trial, those who had taken the CBC online challenge reported that they had lost over 86,000 lbs, and three months into the challenge, more than 360,000 lbs had been lost. (If that level of weight loss is sustained over 2011, the challenge will be met.) The clear message to Canadians is that we're fat and not fit, and we need to do something now about our unhealthy lifestyles.

That we are not now "living right" is brought into sharp relief by the CBC reality program *Village on a Diet*, which follows the residents of Taylor, British Columbia. Nearly 60 percent of the town of close to 1,500 is either overweight or obese. Collectively, the townspeople are aiming to lose one ton (2,000 lbs) in 10 weeks. The townspeople are going on a diet, increasing their exercise, and getting healthier, and they are doing this together. Two trainers working with the community subject them to boot-camp regimes not very different from what can be seen weekly on the American reality program, *The Biggest Loser*. Calories are restricted, and instructions in preparing healthy recipes and following better lifestyles are provided. Weight loss is treated like a contest, and there are abundant examples of public degradation ceremonies to which the townspeople are subjected, all "for their own good." Depending on viewers' own circumstances, they are either inspired or entertained. In the end, the residents of Taylor were triumphant. They met the challenge by losing more than one ton. Four months later, the town residents had lost a further 500 lbs. Of course, the focus of *Village on a Diet* and similar efforts to encourage healthy living is not just a strategy to earn television ratings. But will this help tackle what has been described as a global epidemic of overweight and obesity?

Described in 2002 as a public health crisis by the World Health Organization, "globesity" is now seen as a worldwide epidemic (Joint WHO/FAO Expert Consultation on Diet, Nutrition, and the Prevention of Chronic Diseases, 2002). Changes in dietary practices (i.e., too much consumption of high-fat foods, too little consumption of complex carbohydrates) and the tendency toward sedentary lifestyles are now not just common in industrialized countries, they are also being seen in developing countries. Where these dietary practices and lifestyles are found, so too are increasing levels of chronic diseases (e.g., diabetes, hypertension, cardiovascular disease), disability, and premature mortality. The concern is that obesity is an epidemic out of control, and that with a growing number of children who are overweight, the health and economic burdens will be staggering in the future. Obesity specialists decry the prospect that today's children will die of weight-related health problems, and they will die at younger ages than their parents.

The adverse health effects for the individuals who are living with too much weight are numerous and deadly (Dixon & Broom, 2007). Health care systems are struggling to manage obesity and its complications, including heart disease, hypertension, type 2 diabetes, osteoarthritis and related musculoskeletal disorders, some forms of cancer, asthma, and sleep apnea (Lean, 2010). Bariatrics, the branch of medicine that deals with obesity, is a burgeoning field. Health authorities have had to acquire costly infrastructure (e.g., bariatric ambulances, larger beds and examination tables, "wide-bore" MRIs, lifting devices) so that health care workers can provide safe care (for both patients and providers) and appropriate and humane care for people who are overweight or obese.

The costs of obesity to society are also troubling (Muller-Riemenschneider et al., 2010). A 2009 Public Health Agency of Canada report estimated the direct costs of obesity (i.e., health care expenditures) at $1.8 billion (in 2005 dollars) and the indirect costs of obesity (i.e., lost productivity) at $2.5 billion. Similar costs of overweight, as distinct from obesity, have not been measured, but are believed to be substantial. Seldom are the social implications of obesity studied, but they cannot be overlooked. In 1980, DeJong described how obese people are subject to derogation because of their weight. In January 2011, the Canadian Obesity Network hosted the First National Summit on Weight Bias and Discrimination in Toronto. According to Rebecca Puhl, director of research at Yale University's Rudd Center for Food Policy and Obesity, weight discrimination is now as prevalent as racial discrimination. Overweight and obese people experience bias in the workplace, health care settings, schools, interpersonal relationships, and in the media. Weight discrimination can lead to lowered self-esteem, isolation, and despair, and may even exacerbate unhealthy dietary practices. Sadly, there are few sanctions for stigmatizing those who are overweight (Puhl, 2009).

The public discourse about obesity is almost always framed as a crisis. Jia and Lubetkin (2010) report that in the US, obesity is now the leading cause of lost quality-adjusted years of life, outpacing smoking. When Jim Watson was appointed Ontario's Minister of Health in 2005, he asserted that "fat is Ontario's new public health enemy No. 1.... Fat is the new tobacco. I think obesity is the challenge of the 21st century, just as smoking was the challenge of the 20th century" (cited in Gilman, 2008, 15).

In this chapter, I explore overweight and obesity as a new health issue and as an issue related to health care reform, specifically how health care workers' own health (and weight) may be affected by the working conditions and the structure of care within the health system. As in other chapters in this collection, the focus is on the intersection of bodies, social conditions, and social relations. In keeping with the sex- and gender-based approach, I ask: Why is this a women's issue? What are the issues for women? Which women are most affected? Of particular interest is what we can learn from the research on women and health care reform to help explain the trends on overweight and obesity among both patients and providers of health care. How might the structure and conditions of health care (including health care reform) actually contribute to the problem of overweight and obesity among health care workers? And what kinds of changes are required to ensure quality of care for women in their roles as patients and providers? Because so little attention has been focused explicitly on overweight, obesity, and health care, a central aim of this chapter is to ask some new questions, taking into consideration the changing context of health care.

## The Causes and Correlates of Obesity

Obesity is most often framed as an energy imbalance—individuals ingest too much and exercise too little. The solution is presented as simple and straightforward: eat less and exercise more (Shields & Tremblay, 2008). Yet people tend to gain weight for many reasons beyond the simple equation of eating too much food and being too sedentary (e.g., genetics and hormones may play a role, and some health conditions and medical treatments may cause individuals to gain or have difficulty losing weight). As anyone who has tried to lose weight knows, the energy imbalance approach may have scientific validity, but enacting the necessary behaviour changes is often hardly as simple as eating less and exercising more.

In general, solutions to the obesity problem focus mostly on individual responsibility in relation to the energy imbalance approach. A great deal of research is also focused on the social, behavioural, and environmental factors that predispose people to increasing their food intake and/or reducing their physical activity. For example, Dixon and Broom (2007) refer to the various "deadly sins of obesity," including the increasing dependence on commercially produced and "fast" foods and services, stress, the changing dynamics of family life, the increasing trend toward sedentary behaviours (which is exacerbated by leisure time spent in front of televisions and/or computers), and our overdependence on automobiles.

Research on the determinants of health also suggests that attention should be focused on socio-economic factors. Aboriginal peoples, people living in poverty and in rural and remote communities, and individuals who are marginalized from mainstream society by virtue of poverty, ethnicity, or immigration status are more likely to experience food insecurity, a key risk factor in relation to obesity. To experience food insecurity means that one does not have access to safe, nutritious, and adequate food to maintain one's health and well-being. For example, research in Montreal shows that lower socio-economic neighbourhoods are less likely to have access to healthy food outlets, with the consequence that individuals in those neighbourhoods are more likely to make unhealthy food choices (Daniel, Kestens & Paquet, 2009). Similarly, individuals living on the margins of society (however defined) are also less likely to have access to physical activity (Canadian Institute of Health Information [CIHI], 2003).

Some research points to stressful working conditions that may contribute to weight gain (Park, 2009). There may also be structural conditions in the workplace that predispose individuals to overweight and obesity. Studies show that individuals who are employed in jobs that involve shift work—that is, those who do night work and therefore experience disruptions to their circadian rhythms—and individuals who work long hours are all more likely to gain weight (Landsbergis, 2004; Shields, 1999; Zhao & Turner, 2008).

# Overweight and Obesity in Canada

The assessment of weight usually involves using the body mass index (BMI). The measure is calculated as a person's weight (in kilograms) divided by the square of their height (in metres). BMI is a population-based measure, and is not necessarily appropriate for determining whether an individual is underweight or overweight. This measure does not take into account other variables that may be important in accounting for weight (e.g., gender, body type). Nevertheless, it is the standard way in which population weight trends are summarized. Using the BMI, a person is defined as overweight if she or he has a BMI of 25 to 29.9. A person is defined as obese if she or he has a BMI in excess of 30. Normal weight is associated with a BMI in the range of 18.5 to 24.9. A person is deemed to be underweight if she or he has a BMI of less than 18.5. A critique of the BMI as a health indicator is included in the Women and Health Care Reform publication *Bringing Women and Gender into "Healthy Canadians: A Federal Report on Comparable Health Indicators, 2004"* (Willson & Jackson, 2006).

There are many ways of counting the number of people whose weight exceeds what is classified as "normal." Some studies focus on overweight while others focus on obesity. Some studies focus on self-reports of weight and height, while others rely on objective measurements. Depending on what you are measuring and how, a different picture emerges of the extent of overweight and obesity in the population. For example, the Public Health Agency of Canada (PHAC) (2009) estimates that in 2007 the rate of obesity in Canada was 25 percent overall. According to data from the 2009 Canadian Community Health Survey (CCHS), almost 18 percent of the population aged 18 years or older are classified as obese based on self-reported data (Statistics Canada, 2010b). In the 2003 CCHS, 15 percent of the Canadian adult population were classified as obese. Objectively measured data provide a different estimate than self-reported data, but the trend is the same: more Canadian women and men are heavier than at any other time in history. Statistics Canada (2010a) reports that 40 percent of adult men and 30 percent of adult women are overweight based on data collected in the Canadian Health Measures Survey. Among adults, overweight and obesity tend to increase with age, reaching a peak in later mid-life (ages 55–64), and then tend to decline in old age.

Overweight and obesity are common throughout the population, but there are notable patterns in different regions of the country, in different socio-economic groups, and among First Nations, Inuit, and Métis peoples. Obesity is least prevalent in British Columbia and Quebec, and highest in the provinces of Saskatchewan, Manitoba, and in the Atlantic region. The relationship between socio-economic status and obesity is complex, particularly when sex/gender is taken into consideration. For example, Craig and colleagues (2005) report that individuals with the least educational attainment are more likely to be overweight or obese, but that men in higher income groups are more likely to be overweight or obese than their low-income counterparts, while higher income women are less likely to be overweight or obese than their low-income counterparts. Among off-reserve Aboriginal Canadians, the rates of obesity are significantly higher than for non-Aboriginal Canadians. Katzmarzyk (2008) reports that the prevalence of obesity is higher in Aboriginal children and adults than in non-Aboriginal children and adults (15.8 percent versus 8.0 percent, based on data from the 2004 CCHS). Rates of obesity are higher for Aboriginal women than for Aboriginal men (Garriguet, 2008).

These patterns of overweight and obesity mirror various social inequalities in society, and demonstrate that individuals on the margins have the greatest risk and bear the greatest burden of obesity (Lee, 2011). To effect changes to these patterns of risk and burden will require a focus on the social, structural, and environmental determinants of obesity. This will require that we "refocus upstream" and reorient our strategies for dealing with overweight and obesity from their current focus on individual responsibility to the social conditions that encourage less than healthy behaviours and choices (McKinlay, 1979). This is an area that warrants far more attention than it currently gets from researchers who study overweight and obesity.

# Is Weight a Women's Health Issue?

Weight has long been thought of as a women's health issue. It isn't that men are not overweight and obese—in fact, as noted in the last section, 10 percent more men in Canada are overweight than women—but there are gendered dimensions to the experience of weight gain.

A review of research by Kiefer, Rathmanner, and Kunze (2005) points to different levels of nutritional awareness and food literacy among women and men, and different consumption patterns for women and men. For example, men tend to eat more meat, while women eat more vegetables and fruit; men consume more sugar than women; and men consume more alcohol than women. More women restrict their caloric intake than do men. Women are more likely to snack between meals, though their snacks tend to be healthier than the ones chosen by men (i.e., fruit or yogurt for women as opposed to savoury snacks for men). Women more commonly report food cravings (Kiefer et al., 2005). When it comes to physical activity, men's participation rates are much higher than women's (WHO, n.d.). These examples of gender differences in nutritional behaviours and activity levels do not take into consideration other important sources of variation such as class, race/ethnicity, area of residence, and access to food choices.

Another way in which we can consider the gendered dimensions of weight relates to societal perspectives on preferred body forms. Over time and in different societies and cultures, body ideals have changed dramatically. Consider the contrast between Paul Rubens' glorification of full-figured women in the 1600s with our modern glorification and obsession with lean and slender bodies. In today's globalized world, "the idealised thin Western female body [is] *the* body to possess" (Orbach, 2009, 168). In such a context, many girls and women are dissatisfied with their bodies (and their weight, in particular), and this feeling is normal (Marchessault, 2000) and pervasive. According to the Canadian Women's Health Network (2005), 90 percent of women are unhappy about some aspect of their appearance. Weight preoccupation has been reported in girls as young as five (Gilman, 2008). The results of this weight preoccupation include disordered eating (anorexia and bulimia, as well as overweight and obesity), extreme exercising, depression, self-loathing, isolation, and, in extreme cases, suicidal thoughts.

Rhode (2010) asserts that the "beauty bias" in North American society means women pay a higher price for being overweight. They are more likely to be harshly judged and to be viewed as unattractive, affecting their personal (and sexual) relationships, as well as their work-life experiences. Overweight and obese women are more likely to be paid less and to advance in their occupations more slowly. Women's preoccupation with their weight has spawned (some would say it has been caused by) a vast industry that exploits and reinforces women's dissatisfaction with their bodies. Everything from cosmetics to the diet industry to cosmetic surgery offers women a way to emulate or conform to the idealized notion of the female form, no matter how unattainable that goal may be.

Some health conditions are unique, more prevalent, more serious, or require different interventions in women, making a gender analysis critical (Greaves et al., 1999). In the context of overweight and obesity, certain endocrine problems occur only in women (e.g., polycystic ovarian syndrome) and may predispose them to weight gain and other related health problems. Overweight and obesity are risk factors for cardiovascular disease, the leading cause of death in women. Suboptimal management of cardiovascular disease may put women at greater risk of premature mortality. In the past, research on cardiovascular disease and its treatment was based almost exclusively on male patients and their presenting symptoms. Today, more gendered research has led clinicians to treat women differently based on their presenting symptoms, their subjective assessments of pain, etc. Other problems such as osteoarthritis, diabetes, and infertility, to name just a few, are correlated with overweight and obesity, and the issues for women are different in terms of onset and management.

Overweight and obesity is a complex issue. It is important not to essentialize the experience of weight among women, or to conclude that only women have health issues related to weight. Clearly, men also have weight issues (Haslam, 2005; Peixoto Labre, 2005; Weltzin et al., 2005). There are important gender dimensions to overweight, the factors that influence dietary choices and activity levels, and the health consequences. In the following sections, I explore specific ways in which the issue of overweight and obesity is experienced by women patients, and then look at how the structure of health care may be a factor in overweight among health care workers.

## Issues for Women Patients

Research on weight bias and discrimination shows that individuals who are obese are more likely to have negative experiences in the health care system (Wright, 1998; Puhl & Brownell, 2001;

Brown, 2006). In general, health care professionals tend to have negative perceptions of individuals who are overweight, and have been found to hold stereotypic views (e.g., fat patients are lazy, non-compliant, and lack self-control). Some research has raised concerns about the quality of care that overweight and obese patients receive. Overweight and obese patients who feel they are negatively judged because of their weight may avoid accessing care even though their health needs may be very great (Puhl & Brownell, 2001).

Women and Health Care Reform undertook a qualitative study on women's perspectives of the quality of health care in 2003–2004 (see also Chapter 9). The research was designed to document women's encounters with the health care system in their roles as patients, providers, and decision-makers. A total of 145 women from across Canada were interviewed in 25 focus groups about their experiences in the health care system. Included in the study were women who were obese.

This study shows that Canadian women have definite ideas about quality health care: It is women-centred, comprehensive, focused on prevention, integrated, characterized by continuity, and has a long-term focus. In addition, they consider quality care to be accessible, culturally competent, involving a range of providers, holistic, and cognizant of the changing nature of women's roles in society. To a large degree, for the women we interviewed, attention to the process of care and the contexts of women's lives are the keys to quality.

For many of the women we interviewed the attitudes of health care providers were a key obstacle to quality care. The obese women in our study shared experiences that have been corroborated in other studies of weight bias and discrimination. For example, one woman said, "Being overweight my whole life, the only thing the doctors wanted to do was put me on a diet." Even as a young teenager, she reported that she was given amphetamines to suppress her appetite. Another woman said, "You're treated like you're a second-class citizen because of the way you look. Shouldn't I get health care like everybody else should get?" Another woman shared that no matter who the practitioner was (even her dentist), or what the problem was (she suffered from dandruff), the standard line to her was "'You need to lose weight!' It's not funny. You're very definitely treated very differently when you're overweight. It's almost as if every single issue is the weight." The trivialization of health problems, the essentialization of health problems (to their weight), and the feeling of being disrespected were repeated again and again.

The accounts of the women we interviewed serve as a reminder of the problem of weight bias and discrimination, though overweight and obese men do not escape similar maltreatment. This research, and the substantial literature on overweight and obese patients' encounters with the health care system, remind us that quality of care is structurally affected when people are "othered" in their encounters with health care. The results may be compromised health status, avoidance of health care, and increasing marginalization in a society that punishes people for being overweight. There is much to be done to counter the negative stereotypes of people who are overweight and obese (Puhl, 2009).

## The Work and Weight of Health Care Providers

The health care system is a microcosm of the larger society, so it should come as no surprise that some health care providers are themselves overweight or obese. A *New York Times* headline in 2009 read, "When Weight Is the Issue, Doctors Struggle Too" (Klass, 2009). And when Dr. Regina Benjamin was named as the US Surgeon-General by President Barack Obama, Internet chat rooms debated whether a woman "on the heavy side" could be entrusted to serve as an appropriate role model and the leader of the national health agenda.

While there is research on the physical and mental health of health care workers, there have been no systematic studies to determine whether health care workers are more or less heavy than the general population. And while health care professionals may have more information about health and healthy living, they do not always "walk the walk." When the question "Why are nurses so overweight?" was posted on *The Straight Dope*, an internet message board, one respondent wrote, "Maybe obesity is no more common among nurses than it is in the general population, but it sticks out more because we don't expect it. Maybe we unconsciously reason that these are medical professionals—they *shouldn't be* overweight." The judgment that health care workers should maintain healthy weights relates primarily to their involvement in health promotion and education. How, one might ask, can a doctor or nurse who is overweight counsel a patient to lose weight or adopt a healthier lifestyle? Perhaps an overweight nurse would be more compassionate toward a patient who is overweight, or perhaps an overweight doctor might be less likely to admonish a patient about being overweight.

We have little information on the weight of health care professionals since there are few systematic studies of this segment of the workforce. It is useful to consider what we do and don't know. Two issues come to mind. First, what are the factors in the health care system that may make health professionals (particularly women) susceptible to weight gain? And, second, why does this matter for health care workers and their patients?

Health care workers are subject to the same influences and experiences as the population at large. Our personal experiences with food, with family and friends, with stress and coping all shape our everyday lives and our work lives. In addition, as chapters 6, 7, and 8 show, the conditions of caring work have a bearing on how individuals work, the quality of their work lives, and their health and well-being.

In the 2005 National Survey of the Work and Health of Nurses (Shields & Wilkins, 2006), nurses rate their physical health as mostly good, while their assessment of their mental health is less favourable. Nurses also report more problems with back pain and arthritis than do those in the general population. Shields and Wilkins say that about one-third of nurses indicate that their physical health affects their ability to handle their workload. The experience of work stress is common among nurses. Indicators of work stress include high job strain, precarious work, physically demanding workloads, low autonomy, inadequate support from supervisors, poor working relations with physicians, and role overload (Shields & Wilkins, 2006, xv). The rates of absenteeism due to illness or disability among nurses are consistently higher than in other occupations (CIHI, 2002; Shamian et al., 2003).

No Canadian data are available on BMI or specific health conditions for nurses or other health professionals. The Nurses Health Study in the US collected information on BMI (Field et al., 2007; Setty et al., 2007), but this study is not about nurses as nurses; rather, it is a prospective cohort study of middle-aged women. It does not compare the study cohort's BMI to the BMI of the population at large. The Nurses Health Study looks at determinants associated with weight (e.g., physical activity, television viewing times, and the consumption of selected foods and alcohol), and relates these to various health measures (e.g., the incidence of type 2 diabetes, cardiovascular risk factors). Clearly, we should seek to understand in much greater detail all dimensions of nurses' health (including weight) and the health of other women involved in both paid and unpaid care.

What are the factors in health care work that might contribute to overweight and obesity among nurses? As noted, a number of working conditions are highly correlated with obesity, including shift work, long hours, high job demands/low job control, and conflicts between work and family roles. All of these characteristics are typical of the working lives of nurses. The typical nurse works 12-hour shifts, which usually spill over well past the time period for which they are paid. Many nurses work night shifts, and experience disruptions in their sleep. Given staff shortages, nurses have little downtime during their shifts. All of these aspects of their work may lead to less than optimal nutritional habits and lifestyle practices. In the context of health care reform, nurses may have limited control over their working conditions. And as many nurses are also involved in family care responsibilities, they are routinely involved in juggling double duty at work and at home.

Feminist political economy reminds us that the relations of work, the gendered relations of work and care, the personal and structural factors in women's lives all influence both work and health. Much more information is needed to understand how nurses' caring work affects their health and well-being, and the specific ways in which the structures and relations affect health and health behaviours.

The health of health care workers is important to those workers; it is also important to their patients and to the system as a whole. It is well established that work-related injuries are common among nurses and other health care workers. Back injuries, in particular, are prevalent among nurses (CIHI, 2002). Back pain and injuries are also common in individuals who are overweight. Research on work, weight, and health may give us an important perspective on issues related to patient and worker safety.

## Concluding Remarks

The issue of overweight and obesity is a complex health issue that has been studied extensively, yet many questions remain. Although we know many things about women and weight, we still have relatively little information about overweight and obese patients' experiences in the health care system. We know even less about health care providers' experiences of overweight and obesity both in terms of their own experiences, and how they provide care to individuals who are overweight or obese. Given that more and more Canadians are counted among the population that are overweight, we would do well to develop a better understanding of this phenomenon. Doing so through a gender lens will help ensure that strategies to deal with overweight and obesity are appropriate for women as well as men.

# References

Brown, I. (2006). Nurses' attitudes towards adult patients who are obese: Literature review. *Journal of Advanced Nursing* 53(2), 221–232.

Canadian Institute of Health Information [CIHI]. (2002). *Canada's health care providers.* Ottawa: CIHI.

Canadian Institute of Health Information [CIHI]. (2003). *Obesity in Canada: Identifying policy priorities (proceedings of a roundtable, Ottawa, ON, June 23–24, 2003).* Ottawa: CIHI.

Canadian Women's Health Network (Body Image and the Media). (2005). Retrieved from http://www.cwhn.ca/node/40776

Craig, C.L., Cameron, C. & Bauman, A. (2005). *Socio-demographic and lifestyle correlates of obesity: Technical report on the secondary analyses using the 2000–2001 Canadian community health survey.* Ottawa: CIHI.

Daniel, M., Kestens, Y. & Paquet, C. (2009). Demographic and urban form correlates of healthful and unhealthful food availability in Montreal, Canada. *Canadian Journal of Public Health* 100(3), 189–193.

DeJong, W. (1980). The stigma of obesity: The consequences of naive assumptions concerning the causes of physical deviance. *Journal of Health and Social Behavior* 21, 75–87.

Dixon, J. & Broom, D.H. (Eds.). (2007). *The seven deadly sins of obesity: How the modern world is making us fat.* Sydney: University of New South Wales Press.

Field, A.E., Willett, W.C., Lissner, L. & Colditz, G.A. (2007). Dietary fat and weight gain among women in the nurses' health study. *Obesity* 15(4), 967–976.

Garriguet, D. (2008). Obesity and the eating habits of the Aboriginal population. *Health Reports* 19(1), 1–15. Statistics Canada Catalogue 82-003.

Gilman, S.L. (2008). *Fat: A cultural history of obesity.* Cambridge: Polity Press.

Greaves, L., Hankivsky, O., Amaratunga, C., Ballem, P., Chow, D., De Koninck, M., Grant, K.R., Lippman, A., Maclean, H., Maher, J., Messing, K. & Vissandjée, B. (1999). *CIHR 2000: Sex, gender, and women's health*. Commissioned position paper submitted to the Social Sciences and Humanities Research Council and the Canadian Health Services Research Foundation.

Haslam, D. (2005). Gender-specific aspects of obesity. *Journal of Men's Health and Gender* 2(2), 179–185.

Jia, H. & Lubetkin, E.I. (2010). Trends in quality-adjusted life-years lost contributed by smoking and obesity. *American Journal of Preventive Medicine 38*(2), 138–144.

Joint WHO/FAO Expert Consultation on Diet, Nutrition, and the Prevention of Chronic Diseases. (2002). *Diet, nutrition, and the prevention of chronic diseases: Report of a joint WHO/FAO expert consultation*. WHO technical report series 916. Geneva: World Health Organization.

Katzmarzyk, P.T. (2008). Obesity and physical activity among Aboriginal Canadians. *Obesity 16*(1), 184–190.

Kiefer, I., Rathmanner, T. & Kunze, M. (2005). Eating and dieting differences in men and women. *Journal of Men's Health and Gender* 2(2), 194–201.

Klass, P. (2009). When weight is the issue, doctors struggle too. *New York Times*, July 21. Retrieved from http://www.nytimes.com/2009/07/21/health/21klas.html

Landsbergis, P. (2004). Long work hours, hypertension, and cardiovascular disease. *Cadernos de Saude Publica (Reports in Public Health)* 20(6), 1746–1748.

Lean, M. (2010). Health consequences of overweight and obesity in adults. In D. Crawford, R.W. Jeffery, K. Ball & J. Brug (Eds.), *Obesity epidemiology: From aetiology to public health* (2nd ed.) (pp. 43–58). New York: Oxford University Press.

Lee, H. (2011). Inequality as an explanation for obesity in the United States. *Sociology Compass 5*(3) 215–232.

Marchessault, G. (2000). One mother and daughter approach to resisting weight preoccupation. In B. Miedema, J.M. Stoppard & V. Anderson, *Women's bodies, women's lives: Health, well-being, and body image* (pp. 203–226). Toronto: Sumach Press.

McKinlay, J.B. (1979). A case for refocusing upstream: The political economy of illness. In J.G. Jaco (Ed.), *Patients, physicians, and illness:*

*A sourcebook in behavioral science and health* (pp. 9–25). New York: Free Press.

Muller-Riemenschneider, F., Reinhold, T., von Schulzendorff, A. & Willich, S.N. (2010). Health economic burden of obesity—an international perspective. In D. Crawford, R.W. Jeffery, K. Ball & J. Brug (Eds.), *Obesity epidemiology: From aetiology to public health* (2nd ed.) (pp. 74–88). New York: Oxford University Press.

Orbach, S. (2009). *Bodies*. New York: Picador.

Park, J. (2009). Obesity on the job. *Perspectives* . February 14–22. Statistics Canada Catalogue no. 75-001-X.

Peixoto Labre, M. (2005). The male body ideal: Perspectives of readers and non-readers of fitness magazines. *Journal of Men's Health and Gender* 2(2), 223–229.

Public Health Agency of Canada (PHAC). (2009). Obesity in Canada—snapshot. Ottawa: PHAC. Retrieved from http://www.phac-aspc.gc.ca

Puhl, R. (2009). Bias and stigma weigh heavily on efforts to overcome obesity. *Conduit* 3(3), 4.

Puhl, R. & Brownell, K.D. (2001). Bias, discrimination, and obesity. *Obesity Research* 9(12), 788–805.

Rhode, D.L. (2010). *The beauty bias: The injustice of appearance in life and law*. New York: Oxford University Press.

Seidell, J.C. (2010). Prevalence and trends in adult obesity in affluent countries. In D. Crawford, R.W. Jeffery, K. Ball & J. Brug (Eds.), *Obesity epidemiology: From aetiology to public health* (2nd ed.) (pp. 17–26). New York: Oxford University Press.

Setty, A.R., Curhan, G. & Choi, H.K. (2007). Obesity, waist circumference, weight change, and the risk of psoriasis in women: Nurses' health study II. *Archives of Internal Medicine 167*(15), 1670–1675.

Shamian, J., O'Brien-Pallas, L., Thomson, D., Alksnis, C. & Kerr, M.S. (2003). Nurse absenteeism, stress, and workplace injury: What are the contributing factors and what can/should be done about it? *International Journal of Sociology and Social Policy* 23(8/9), 81–103.

Shields, M. (1999). Long working hours and health. *Health Reports 11*(2), 33–48. Statistics Canada Catalogue no. 82-003.

Shields, M. & Tremblay, M.S. (2008). Sedentary behaviour and obesity.

*Health Reports 19*(2), 19–28. Statistics Canada Catalogue no. 82-003.

Shields, M. & Wilkins, K. (2006). *Findings from the 2005 national survey of the work and health of nurses.* Statistics Canada Catalogue no. 83-003-XIE. Ottawa: Statistics Canada.

Statistics Canada. (2009). Overweight and obese adults (self-reported), 2009. Retrieved from http://www.statcan.gc.ca/pub/82-625-x/2010002/article/11255-eng.htm

Statistics Canada. (2010a). Body composition of Canadian adults, 2007 to 2009. *Health Fact Sheets.* Statistics Canada Catalogue no. 82-625-X. Ottawa: Statistics Canada.

Statistics Canada. (2010b). *The Daily,* June 15, 2010. Retrieved from http://www.statcan.gc.ca/daily-quotidien/100615/dq100615b-eng.htm

Weltzin, T.E., Weisensel, N., Franczyk, D., Burnett, K., Klitz, C. & Bean, P. (2005). Eating disorders in men: Update. *Journal of Men's Health and Gender 2*(2), 186–193.

Willson, K. & Jackson, B.E. (2006). *Bringing women and gender into "Healthy Canadians: A federal report on comparable health indicators, 2004."* Winnipeg: National Coordinating Group on Health Care Reform and Women.

World Health Organization. (n.d.). *Physical activity and women (factsheet).* Retrieved from http://www.who.int/dietphysicalactivity/factsheet_women/en/index.html

Wright, J. (1998). Female nurses' perceptions of acceptable female body size: An exploratory study. *Journal of Clinical Nursing 7*, 307–315.

Zhao, I. & Turner, C. (2008). The impact of shift work on people's daily health habits and adverse health outcomes. *Australian Journal of Advanced Nursing 25*(3), 8–22.

CHAPTER 12

# An Unfinished Revolution

PAT ARMSTRONG

Women and Health Care Reform (WHCR) has established innovative models for research, for knowledge creation, and for knowledge sharing, models that have been copied within Canada and
around the world. We have understood the creation and sharing
of knowledge both as collective processes and as overlapping
ones. We have been, from the beginning, committed to collaborative and interdisciplinary work in keeping with our mandate.
Face-to-face meetings were essential to our process. These meetings were critical in part because we were dispersed across the
country in various centres and involved in other multiple work
demands. But the meetings were also fundamental to the development of new ideas, new approaches, and new means of knowledge sharing. Coordination and integration of research required
shared rather than individual effort. So did the identification of
gaps in research, policies, and practices, and in the development
of strategies both to address them and to use knowledge to effect
change. In these meeting ideas were presented, challenged, modified, and acted upon; research was initiated and analysis written;
workshops were organized and policy forums developed; and the

format for popular pieces was created and implemented. In these meetings we developed relationships of trust that allowed us to work together quickly and effectively, based on our shared histories and knowledge of each other's strengths.

Together we have explored many issues from women's perspectives, seeking always to be sensitive to the differential impact of policies and practices. In doing so, we have frequently sought to anticipate and even prompt issues in an effort to shape policy in the making. We have brought together researchers, policy-makers, and practitioners, using our background documents as a platform for prompting not only more research and awareness of research but policy change. We have worked in and with a wide range of community and government agencies. Over the 13 years of our existence, this work was made possible by funding from Health Canada, although our work did not necessarily represent Health Canada's policies. The funding allowed us to develop an effective and efficient way of operating, based on a history of collaboration, trust, and interdisciplinary cross-fertilization.

This history, this interdisciplinarity, this familiarity, this connection to communities, and this experience with research and knowledge sharing made us nimble and able to respond quickly and on the basis of evidence. One example relates to the Royal Commission on the Future of Health Care in Canada (2002). We organized a meeting for the day the report was to be released, adding to our numbers two people with expertise to complement our own. Together and within hours of the report being made public, we developed a preliminary gender-based analysis and wrote a press release that was picked up across the country. We then went home to write up individually a more extensive, chapter-by-chapter analysis, which was quickly published as *Reading Romanow* (National Coordinating Group on Health Care Reform and Women, 2003). We used *Reading Romanow* at subsequent policy meetings and had the satisfaction of hearing those involved in producing the Romanow Commission report acknowledge that it was a mistake to ignore the issues for women. Invited to our workshop on ancillary workers in health services, a senior member of the Romanow research team said he came because he had learned valuable lessons from our analysis.

A second example is what we call our elevator paper. Madeline Boscoe, then executive director of Canadian Women's Health Network (CWHN) and a long-serving member of WHCR, happened to share an elevator with a colleague of the federal advisor on wait times. Madeline asked what the advisor was doing about gender, and the conversation led to an invitation to write an appendix to the advisor's report (Postl, 2006). The time frame was short and we were able to respond to the invitation because we had a team with expertise in gender-based analysis, a team accustomed to working together. The result was not only an appendix. References to the importance of gender-based analysis were integrated into the text of the report itself.

This book is intended as a legacy project from a group that has made a difference in policy, research, and practice. It updates issues from those 13 years of work and demonstrates that these issues continue to be critical for women. It does not include all the issues we have tackled. For example, we have produced materials intended to guide those working in emergency preparedness and disaster response to anticipate the ways that gender matters (Enarson, 2009). There are also many issues we have not taken up in our years of work. One example is the global context of health care. The growth of reproductive tourism, with women travelling across the globe to seek assistance in becoming pregnant, cries out for a gender analysis; so does the development in Canada of what Arlie Russell Hochschild (2000) calls "global care chains," which sees women from low-income countries leaving their own families at home in order to care for the families of Canadians. The use of technology to substitute for health care workers in the home and in the hospital has not been explored from a gender perspective. These are just three of many matters that we have not had time to address. Yet all of the issues we consider here are still relevant. In spite of the evidence clearly demonstrating that gender matters, that gender must always be part of the question, and that all health care issues are women's issues, the overwhelming majority of research on health care reform fails to take gender into account.

At least as important as the lack of gender-based analysis are the gaps among evidence, policies, and practices. For instance, there is plenty of evidence to show that keeping health care facilities clean is critical to health and requires skills that are quite different from those involved in cleaning hotels, yet we continue to contract out hospital housekeeping services and to dismiss cleaning as unskilled work any woman can do (Armstrong, Armstrong & Scott-Dixon, 2008).

In short, like other women's work, the work of applying a gender-based analysis in research, policy, and practice is "never done." It is work that is never completed and, even in areas where we have made significant progress, requires constant monitoring and vigilance to ensure we do not lose what we have gained. Nevertheless, the work will no longer be done by the collective known as Women and Health Care Reform because our funding ends in 2011, reflecting new government priorities and approaches to funding. Our materials will continue to be mounted on the CWHN website and our popular pieces will still be available through CWHN. We hope this book prompts others to continue and expand the work we have only just begun.

# References

Armstrong, P., Armstrong, H. & Scott-Dixon, K. (2008). *Critical to care: The invisible women in health services.* Toronto: University of Toronto Press.

Enarson, E. (2009). *Not just victims: Women in emergencies and disasters.* Winnipeg: Women and Health Care Reform.

Hochschild, A.R. (2000). Global care chains and emotional surplus value. In W. Hutton & A. Giddens (Eds.), *On the Edge: Living with*

*Global capitalism.* pp. 130–146. New York: Norton.

National Coordinating Group on Health Care Reform and Women. (2003). *Reading Romanow.* Toronto: National Network on Environments and Women's Health.

Postl, B. (2006). *Final report of the federal advisor on wait times.* Ottawa: Health Canada.

Royal Commission on the Future of Health Care. (2002). *Building on values: The future of health care in Canada. Final report.* Ottawa: Commission on the Future of Health Care in Canada.

# The Charlottetown Declaration on the Right to Care

## NOVEMBER 10, 2001

In Charlottetown in November 2001, 55 experts from the academic, policy, and caregiver communities gathered to discuss research and policy on women and home care. With the assistance of documents that brought together the research that examined gender in relation to home and community care, they assessed existing literature, demonstrating that:

- women are the majority of unpaid and paid care providers, and of care receivers;
- women face different expectations, have fewer and different resources than men;
- women provide more demanding care, work longer hours, and have more responsibility;
- women providing care often end up in poor health;
- women's lives and plans are more disrupted, and negatively so, by caregiving;
- women have more supportive networks, but these too may be a source of conflict;

- women are rewarded by caregiving, although inadequate resources limit rewards and make it harder to care;
- women with care needs receive fewer hours of care than men;
- women from immigrant, refugee, and visible minority communities face racism, language, and cultural barriers;
- First Nations, Inuit, and Métis women in particular are disadvantaged in giving and receiving care;
- women receiving and giving care are subject to violence and other physical risks.

Those participating in the workshop agreed that we now have sufficient evidence to transform research into policy and practice. They decided to spend most of their time on this urgent task. On the basis of this work, they:

- called for legislative initiatives;
- created networks for future research and for policy exchange and development;
- identified a research agenda to fill gaps, to use existing data sources more effectively, and to develop models for assessment and change;
- supported research and policy that recognizes the traditional practices and activities of First Nations, Inuit, and Métis;
- considered the basis for a strategy that recognizes, values, and supports unpaid caregiving.

In turn, the workshops and plenary discussions led toward a consensus on the fundamental principles that should be the basis for such a strategy. These were codified into *The Charlottetown Declaration on the Right to Care*.

*The Charlottetown Declaration on the Right to Care* begins by stating that "The right to care is a fundamental human right." This means that "Canadian society has a collective responsibility to ensure universal entitlement to public care throughout life." Such care must be provided "without discrimination as to gender, ability, age, physical location, sexual orientation, socioeconomic and family status or ethno-cultural origin."

Care is thus understood as a public good rather than as a consumer one, and every effort must be made to make care accessible in ways that recognize both different needs and existing discriminatory practices.

The research makes it clear that there are a number of components necessary in order to support this right.

According to the Declaration, the right to care requires the following:

*First, access to a continuum of services and supports:* Our public system began initially by financing hospitals and then moved on to pay for physicians. But the Hall Royal Commission that led to medicare clearly understood an effective and efficient public system had to provide a full range of coordinated services and supports, including public home care. Indeed, the commission saw the financing of hospitals and doctors as merely the first step because only with a continuum of services would people receive care at the most appropriate level, move easily from one service to another, and avoid costly duplication. Those not using the services often still need public supports such as respite care, equipment, training, and an opportunity to exchange information with others. Such services and supports must be culturally sensitive, taking into account the particular practices and preferences of those involved in the care relationship.

*Second, appropriate conditions:* Whether care is provided at home or in a facility, it is necessary to provide conditions that meet the needs of care recipients and care providers. We know that health is determined by culture, physical and social environment, social support, security, gender, economic and educational resources, and coping skills, as well as by biology, genetic makeup, and health services. These all count in the provision of care, and some are even more important, given the fragility of people who are ill or who have a disability. Homes are not necessarily "havens in a heartless world," and hospitals can be dangerous to the health of patients and providers if conditions do not meet their particular needs or ignore the determinants of health.

*Third, the choice to receive or not receive, or to provide or not to provide unpaid care:* Care involves both the person who gives care and the person who receives care. Both need choices about who provides care and about what care is provided. Women "conscripted" into care, as the prime minister's National Forum on Health was told, themselves end up in poor health and often provide poor care. Women who need care may not want to receive such care from relatives conscripted into service. At the same time, many want to provide care or to receive such help from relatives, but they need help to do so. Public care should provide alternatives in ways that offer a genuine choice for both in the care relationship.

*Fourth, there is no assumption of unpaid care:* Care is not a choice if it is assumed that families in general, and women in particular, are willing and able to provide care. Many lack the skills, other resources, or desire to give or receive unpaid care. This is particularly the case as the majority of women must rely on having income from paid work and as more of the work sent home requires complex treatment. At the same time, unpaid care may not be possible without necessary supports and future planning to ensure that those who do undertake unpaid care work are not penalized now or in the future.

*Fifth, access to reasonable alternatives and sufficient information:* The right to care requires not only a choice about providing or receiving care, but a choice about how and where care is provided. For many, but not all, home may be the best place for care. For some, but not many, facilities may best serve their needs. Such alternatives must be available to ensure appropriate and cultur- ally sensitive care. Moreover, reliable, accessible information on the benefits and problems with alternatives and on how to access them, as well as on how to give and receive care, is a necessary component in a public care system.

To ensure the right to care, *care must be understood as essential,* something we must as a country provide. While we have choices about how, when, and where to provide care, we do not have a choice about whether to provide care to those who need it. We can- not leave people without necessary care. Care must also be under- stood as *an interdependent relationship.* It is not simply about what one person does to or for another, but rather about an exchange that involves two people. This exchange involves *skilled work,* not something that women do naturally by virtue of having female bodies. It requires education, training, and experience to care. Care is at the same time *multidimensional,* involving all aspects of those involved in the relationship. It includes everything from feeding, bathing, and hugging to injecting, chatting, and intubat- ing. And, finally, care is necessarily *diverse,* both because people are different and because they not only have different needs, but different ways their culture and experience say these needs must be addressed.

Such care should be:

*Equitable:* Equitable care does not mean the same care for every- one, but rather a fair distribution of care based on assessed needs. It also means, as the *Canada Health Act* puts it, that care is provided under "uniform terms and conditions."

*Accessible:* Again we can take direction from the *Canada Health Act,* which says that necessary services must be provided in a manner that "does not impede or preclude, either directly or indirectly" access to care. This includes user fees or other charges that can undermine the right to care.*Available:* The *Canada Health Act* recognizes that care must be there in order to be accessible. The right to care has no meaning if there are no services or if services involve long trips and considerable delays.

*Continuous:* Care requires the assurance that it will be there, a smooth transition from service to service, and a range of services that can respond to changing health needs.

*Responsive and transparent:* Care should reflect the particular needs of the individual, responding to these in ways that recognize the specificity of each person giving and receiving care. Decisions about care and the means of accessing care need to be clear and accessible. This includes decisions about what care is publicly provided and what is not.

*Incorporate diversity:* Responsive care is care that also recognizes cultural, regional, age, and gender diversity, as well as differences related to sexual orientation, and socio-economic and family status. Particular attention must be paid to traditional practices and activities of First Nations, Inuit, and Métis.

*Participatory:* Both those providing and those receiving care should be involved in decisions about how, when, where, and by whom care is provided. Citizens in general should also have a say in how the system is constructed.

*Enforceable:* It is not enough to set out the principles for the right to care. It is also necessary to put mechanisms in place to ensure that these rights are protected through the provision of services and supports of the sort that protect this right.

*Standards-based:* Although it is important to respond to individual needs and to allow individuals to participate in deciding about care, it is also necessary to have standards for care based on evidence about efficacy. Evidence should provide guidelines for providers and standards against which care can be compared.

*Publicly administered:* There are clear benefits to a publicly administered health care system in terms of both cost savings and coordination. A publicly administered system is also easier to hold accountable to citizens.

*Respectful:* Care is about individuals with preferences, feelings, experience, minds, and histories. Care should respect each individual and always be provided in ways we would like care provided for ourselves.

These rights to care must be viewed through lenses that recognize the importance of gender analysis, diversity, interdependence between paid and unpaid care, and linkages among social, medical, and economic programs.

# Index

ability/disability, home care and, 151–52
Aboriginal Health Transition Fund (AHTF), 154
Aboriginal peoples:
caregiving as an honour among, 147;
illness rates among, 147;
life expectancy of, 147;
overweight/obesity and, 269, 271–72;
policies and programs for primary and home care for, 154–55. *See also* First Nations; Inuit; Métis
Aboriginal women:
access to residential LTC for, 118;
aggregate discussion of, 148;
gendered and culturally prescribed roles of, 147;
home care and, 146–48;
isolation and, 147, 207;
low-paying jobs of, 147;
maternal mortality among, 88, 101;
rural isolation of, 147;
underrepresentation of in nursing, 177
abortion, private health insurance and, 249
abuse:
emotional, 202;
male nurses and, 202;
private health insurance and history of, 246;
risk of in home care, 152. *See also* discrimination; violence
access to health care services:
Aboriginal women and, 118;
barriers to, 40, 46, 50, 51, 252;
*Canada Health Act* and, 235–36;
collaborative care and, 44;
doctors and, 168, 174;
enhancement of, 42–43;
equality of, 115, 239;
ethnic minorities and, 129, 148;
inequities in, 11, 250–51;